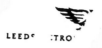

Basic Principles of Auditory Assessment

Basic Principles of Auditory Assessment

Maureen Hannley, Ph.D.
Department of Speech and Hearing Science
Arizona State University

Taylor & Francis Ltd
London

Published by
Taylor & Francis Ltd., 4 John Street, London WC1N 2ET

First published by
College-Hill Press, 4284 41 Street, San Diego, CA 92105

Copyright © 1986 by College-Hill Press, Inc.

Library of Congress Cataloging-in-Publication Data
Main entry under title:

Hannley, Maureen, 1942–
    Basic principles of auditory assessment.

    Includes bibliographies and index.
    1. Hearing disorders—Diagnosis.   2. Audiometry. I. Title. (DNLM: 1.
Hearing–physiology.   2. Hearing Tests–methods.   3. Hearing
Disorders–diagnosis.
WV 272 H245c)
RF294.H34 1986 617.8'9 85-30865

ISBN 0-316-343412

British Library Cataloging in Publication Data

Hannley, Maureen
    Clinical assessment of auditory function: basic procedures.
    1. Audiometry
    I. Title
    617.8'9'0287 RF294

ISBN 0-85066-604-X

This edition not for sale in the American continent

Printed in the United States of America

To my teachers and models,
Dr. James Jerger
Dr. Charles I. Berlin

CONTENTS

Preface

Almost half a century ago, a young speech pathologist named Dr. Raymond Carhart was overwhelmed with the number of veterans returning from World War II with significant hearing impairments. He devoted the rest of his career to the study of hearing disorders, hearing assessment, and procedures for hearing aid evaluation. His pioneering work at the Deshon Veterans Administration Hospital, and later at Northwestern University, resulted in the emergence of audiology as a profession, and earned for Dr. Carhart the title "Father of Audiology." The tools available for assessing auditory function were few and, by today's standards, rudimentary. Other scientists soon, however, began to enter the new field, bringing with them specialized knowledge about auditory anatomy and physiology, psychological and physiological acoustics, and engineering.

Armed with an appreciation of normal auditory function and psychophysical methods, these early workers—Carhart, Reger, Davis, Hood, Fairbanks, Jerger, and Owens—played dual roles as clinicians and researchers while developing new methods of assessment. Because there were no "objective" tests in use at that time, the accuracy of clinical hearing tests depended in large part on the clinician's ability to observe the patient, to "read" the tests, and to use inferential reasoning about their significance. There was, in short, a lot of art to the new science of audiology.

Tests grew more sophisticated and more numerous. At the same time, enormous advances in electronic technology and computer science took place. Suddenly (it seemed) there were complex two-channel audiometers with phase-locking and logic circuits, electroacoustic impedance bridges and electroacoustic admittance meters, averaging computers for evoked potentials, electronystagmographs, and phase shifters.

With all these powerful tools at hand, the arts of skilled patient observation and inferential thinking had a tendency to recede into the background and to be replaced with an emphasis on the technological and procedural aspects of assessment. Equipment has become ever more automatic—"user-oriented"—to the extent that it sometimes relieves the user of all responsibility for knowing what he or she is doing.

Today's students are faced with a broad array of instruments, procedures, and protocols as they prepare for a career in audiology—so many, it seems, that the course of study must be dominated by learning how to test, and not how to observe, how to listen, or how to figure things out. The relevance of basic science courses in anatomy and physiology of the auditory system and hearing science to testing methods often becomes unclear.

There are two related issues that have developed from the technological revolution in audiology. The first has been discussed by Tobin (1978). He characterized two approaches to auditory assessment: the *disordered systems* approach and the *disordered functions* approach. Historically, the disordered systems approach has received the most emphasis in the search to define the site of an auditory disorder, and it relies heavily on technology. The disordered functions approach requires no less rigorous testing methods, but in this case the information is used to assess the effects of hearing impairment on communication and to plan a program of habilitation. The role of the clinician changes from a provider of information to a provider of assistance.

The two approaches, however, are interdependent rather than independent. The goal of any diagnostic procedure is to learn the nature of a problem so that an appropriate management plan can be implemented. But the success of a management plan depends in large measure on the accuracy of the diagnosis and on the clinician's ability to select a combination of assessment procedures uniquely suited to the problem under investigation.

To make a truly informed selection, the clinician must know how each test works, what aspect of auditory function the procedure tests, the meaning of various results, how reliable and valid the procedures are in identifying a problem, and what the results mean in terms of "real life" communicative function. Moreover, this deep an understanding enables the clinician to communicate more effectively with the patient as the results of the evaluation are presented—not in jargon or highly technical language, but at a level most meaningful and relevant to the patient. The same mastery of tests assists communication with the patient's family, teachers, physician, employer, and other significant persons.

The second issue, as already noted, is that beginning students are often so busy learning the mechanics of the profession that they may not have time to think about what it all means. Ultimately, they are limited to a disordered systems approach, and sometimes a mechanical one at that. My increasing concern over this issue has led me to write this book.

PURPOSES OF THE BOOK

This is a book about the principles and philosophies underlying the clinical assessment of auditory function. It is not a "cookbook" with step-by-step procedures, nor is it a comprehensive review of the literature that has shaped clinical procedures. There are other books that fulfill those functions quite well.

The process of hearing assessment gains significance from an understanding of its basis in physiological and phychological acoustics. Stated more simply, there are logical reasons why auditory tests turn out as they do; one aim of this book is to help the reader develop an understanding—not a rote memory—of basic auditory tests, as well as an appreciation of deductive logic used to interpret and use the results of those tests.

A project of this sort could become unreasonably lengthy if it attempted to cover all aspects of auditory testing and their foundations in the basic sciences. Therefore, I have limited the material in three respects. First, the text is directed to the level of a student who has completed coursework in auditory anatomy and physiology, basic hearing science, and psychophysical methods. Second, the material is limited to the assessment of adults and children of school age or older. Pediatric audiology is a very special and complex area, requiring unique observation skills, test techniques, and perseverance. It would be inappropriate to imply, by failing to impose this limitation, that the same procedures are applicable across all age groups. Third, this book is devoted to a consideration of *basic* techniques—those that would be used in an initial evaluation—rather than those used in a search for the "site of lesion" or in selecting a hearing aid.

The chapters have been arranged in chronological order, that is, the order in which I believe the procedures would be used most efficiently in the clinical situation. Thus, equipment calibration and listening checks begin the clinical sections, followed by the case history, immittance audiometry, pure tone audiometry and masking, speech audiometry, and interpretation of patterns of test results. As you will see, adherence to this sequence permits a series of logical decisions and hypothesis testing to take place during the assessment.

A rather lengthy discussion of some basic principles underlying acoustic immittance measures appears in Chapter 4. Although such a discussion may seem to be out of step with the highly clinical tone of the rest of the book, I have included it on the basis of my strong conviction that the responsible use and interpretation of physiological measures of auditory function demands a thorough understanding of the physical and acoustic principles governing such measurements. Throughout the book references have been kept to a minimum to encourage the flow of discussion. Questions for study and discussion, as well as suggested general reading, are provided at the end of most chapters.

This book was written for use as a teaching tool. For that reason I have dedicated it to two persons—Dr. James Jerger and Dr. Chuck Berlin—who are internationally recognized as teachers and leaders in clinical audiology, and who have been most influential in my own career as a student, practitioner, and teacher of audiology.

Certain other individuals have contributed to the making of this book in such significant ways that I must acknowledge them by name. Dr. Sadanand Singh planted the idea of a book on clinical assessment in my mind, encouraged its development, and extended unwavering patience and kindness to me throughout the often rocky course of its preparation. Professor Mark P. Haggard permitted me to spend six months studying and writing at the Institute of Hearing Research in Nottingham, England and, with the rest of the laboratory members, gave generously of time, materials, and friendship during that time. Drs. Quentin Summerfield and Kathleen Horner were especially gracious and helpful in every way. At the time I was enjoying the English countryside, Dr. Marjorie Leek was teaching my classes (as well as her own) at Arizona State University, a favor above the call of mere colleagueship.

Among those who gave freely of their time to read all or part of the manuscript and to offer salient, thoughtful, and always tactful advice for its improvement were Patricia Ehret, Geri Burkett, Dr. Wendell Todd, and Dr. Robert Maresca. In addition, the manuscript was read and critiqued very candidly by members of my class in Methods of Audiometry at Arizona State University. Ingrid Cedar helped with library research.

I have relied to an extraordinary extent on the advice and support given me by two very special friends, Professor Michael Dorman, and Dr. Susan Jerger. Each has known what to say and what to do to encourage and prod me through the rough times. Any credit that this book may bring I share freely and gratefully with all those mentioned; responsibility for errors or omissions is mine alone.

Chapter 1

Introduction

The test battery is the foundation of responsible and effective auditory assessment. No one who has studied the structure and function of the ear could fail to be impressed with its elegant complexity. It is only reasonable, then, to approach auditory assessment with a battery of tests, each of which is selected to focus on a particular level of function, and each of which provides cross-checks to other tests in the battery. The following section focuses on the philosophy of the test battery and the cross-check principle, and on the ways in which the components of a test battery are selected.

PHILOSOPHY OF THE TEST BATTERY

The auditory system can be viewed as a series of components, each with its own distinct function, arranged in a quasi-hierarchical manner from peripheral to central sites. As a signal progresses through the system it is modified and processed in different ways; thus, if it is distorted in some way at a given level, the higher levels will receive a less than optimum signal and the distortion becomes additive, or even multiplicative. Because the greatest signal modifications (resonance, impedance matching, tuning) occur at the peripheral levels, peripheral effects will dominate central effects. For example, functional evidence of an outer or middle ear disorder—loudness attenuation—will be more noticeable to the patient than deficits in two-ear interaction produced by a brain stem disorder. Moreover, auditory processing of simple and complex signals (e.g., pure tones and speech) is affected differentially by disorders at certain levels. This means that different types of signals must be presented under a variety of listening conditions to determine the level at which auditory dysfunction is arising.

These principles have three important implications in auditory assessment. First, auditory dysfunction may result from pathology at one or more levels of the system. If an abnormality appears on a given test, it is necessary to rule out or to identify lower level contributions to the problem before attributing the abnormality exclusively to one site. Second, patients can—and often do—have co-existing disorders at several levels, with the most dominant problem masking clues to the presence of others. A patient with a tympanic membrane perforation, for example, can develop a noise-induced hearing impairment and later be found to have an acoustic neuroma. As is true of the rest of the body, disorder at one level does not bestow immunity to disorders at other levels. Third, the results of a battery of tests contribute information about the auditory processes that are normal as well as those that are abnormal. This information is important in planning management after the diagnostic phase is completed.

The need to approach auditory assessment with a battery of tests designed to screen function at several levels of the auditory system is based on the foregoing three practical considerations. The raison d'être of the test battery, then, is *accountability:* accountability for the interpretation of test results, accountability for identifying all sources, overt and covert, of auditory dysfunction; and accountability for understanding how that dysfunction affects the patient's ability to use and process signals of different levels of complexity.

THE CROSS-CHECK PRINCIPLE

The cross-check principle in audiology, originally outlined by Jerger and Hayes (1976) as a guideline for pediatric assessment, can be viewed as an extension of the test battery approach. The principle is that the results of a single test are never accepted as conclusive proof of the nature or site of auditory disorder without support from at least one additional independent test. The strongest cross-check is provided by "objective" physiological tests, such as immittance audiometry or auditory brain stem responses (ABR), in which the results are independent of the patient's voluntary response.

The most compelling argument for applying the cross-check principle to auditory assessment is that the results of the assessment will have a direct impact on the patient's life. If this statement seems dramatic, consider the consequences of failing to identify profound hearing impairment in a child or, conversely, reporting profound impairment when there is none; counseling a patient that there is no need for a hearing aid or that one would be useless; identifying the type of hearing impairment incorrectly, leading to ineffective medical management; failing to recognize signs of a potentially life-threatening retrocochlear auditory disorder. Inappropriate diagnostic conclusions lead to inappropriate management plans, and the results can be devastating.

The cross-check principle has been used in medicine (and in aviation) for some time. An otolaryngologist, for example, uses a battery of three tuning fork tests (the Weber, the Rinne, and the Bing) to identify and cross check the presence of a middle ear disorder. The error inherent in the tests and in patient response behavior is recognized and the probability of an incorrect diagnosis is minimized when the results of several tests lead to the same conclusion. The cross-check principle has the added advantage that, should the diagnosis be questioned, it can be defended by the results of two or more independent, converging tests.

SELECTION OF A TEST BATTERY

The components of a test battery are selected with five goals in mind. Taken together, the tests should (1) act as a screen for disorders at several levels of the auditory system; (2) provide opportunities for making the appropriate cross-checks; (3) address the patient's primary complaint; (4) provide information relevant to the purpose of the assessment; and (5) establish a uniform data base for purposes of research and inter-subject comparison. The first two goals have been discussed briefly in the context of the previous sections.

When asked, patients can usually offer one major complaint that has led them to seek auditory assessment. Most often the complaint is of decreased hearing, particularly for speech under certain listening conditions. Frequently, however, they are most concerned because of noises in the ear (tinnitus), dizziness, or pain or fullness in the ear. A patient whose chief complaint is inability to understand speech when there is background noise should be tested with a battery that includes at least one measure of speech processing in noise, perhaps at several different signal-to-noise ratios. The other components of the battery would be selected to probe auditory function at several levels to identify the source of the dysfunction, and to determine whether immediate medical referral is indicated. The aim of complaint-oriented test selection is not merely to confirm the patient's report but also to obtain some quantifiable measure that will enable the clinician to make some projections about the social communicative effects of the problem and then to decide the best course of action.

The patient who seeks auditory assessment with a specific complaint usually comes with specific questions in mind as well: "Do I have a hearing loss?" "Do I need a hearing aid?" "What is causing this problem?" "Is my loss great enough to qualify me for disability compensation?" Thus, the clinician should determine what the patient's expectations are at the beginning of the assessment. Some questions cannot be answered directly by an audiologist—for example, diagnosis of a pathological condition or assignment of disability rating—but valuable information can be provided to the appropriate specialist.

If the goal of the evaluation is strictly diagnostic (usually upon medical referral), the test battery will be composed of tests that are the most sensitive and reliable indicants of auditory function in the middle ear, cochlea, eighth (auditory) nerve, brain stem, and temporal lobe. If, on the other hand, the evaluation is to assess the feasibility of a hearing aid, the tests of interest would be those that measure performance at several suprathreshold levels, in quiet and with background noise. The battery would also include measures of loudness discomfort and preferred listening level. Evaluations oriented toward the design of aural rehabilitation programs should include tests that allow an analysis of the types of phonemic identification errors the patient makes at ordinary conversational levels and at amplified levels, and a measure of speechreading ability.

Although the goals of the assessment vary among patients, the basic test battery will include many of the same tests. In most instances, pure tone audiometry is completed, and there is some measure of speech processing. There are many reasons why immittance testing should be *routinely* included, optimally at the beginning of the evaluation. The wealth of information provided by immittance measures is the strongest argument for its inclusion as the first test of an assessment done for any reason. Given these common components, the difference among batteries selected for different reasons lies in the different ways in which the test results are used to answer the pertinent questions. This concept will be elaborated in the sections covering the individual test procedures.

As noted earlier in this chapter, many of the pioneers in audiology served dual roles as clinicians and researchers. They recognized that clinical patients can also be regarded as research subjects. This principle has led to the recognition and description of patterns of test results that are characteristic of different forms of auditory disorders. When the same basic set of tests is administered to thousands of patients, important information emerges: patterns of test results can be identified and related to the ways in which pathological conditions affect auditory function; the diagnostic efficiency of various tests can be demonstrated; and the ways that test results are interrelated become clear. This principle has been exemplified in the work of Drs. James and Susan Jerger. By adopting the philosophy that each clinical patient represents an opportunity to learn more about auditory function and dysfunction, the Jergers have made major and lasting contributions to the field of audiology.

An important consideration in the selection of a test battery is the amount of time available for the entire patient contact. In a busy medical office, patients may be scheduled at 15 minute intervals; in a specialized university or hospital setting, one to two hours might be allocated to complex procedures. The clinician should have well in mind the length of time each test requires; added to that is the time anticipated for counseling and direct patient contact. If a limited period of time is available for the initial contact, the test battery will be made up of procedures that yield the most reliable information in the shortest time. In today's world of cost efficiency, accountability, and rising health care costs, the cliche "Time is money" takes on added significance. The diagnostic and time efficiency of components of the basic test battery are discussed later in this book in the chapter on test interpretation.

A fundamental assumption underlying auditory assessment is that the tools necessary to carry out the assessment are available and in good working order. For this reason, regular listening checks and output calibration of all clinical equipment should be made a part of the clinic routine. The next chapter will discuss these procedures.

STUDY QUESTIONS

1. What is meant by the "cross-check principle"?
2. Why is a battery of tests necessary in auditory assessment?
3. How does accountability apply to selection of a test battery?
4. What are some advantages of applying the cross-check principle? Some disadvantages?
5. What goals guide the clinician in selecting a test battery?

Chapter 2

Calibration of Test Equipment

Prior to the development of the electric audiometer in the 1920s, the tools for assessing hearing were relatively simple: tuning forks; pocket or wristwatches; spoken or whispered voice. Such tools, although easy to use, yielded relatively gross and often quite variable information about a patient's hearing. Calibration, in the sense of comparing an output signal to a criterion, did not exist. When audiometers were invented, their use was generally confined to research being conducted on telephone communication systems.

In 1951, the American Standards Association (ASA) adopted as norms for audiometric 0 a set of data on "normal" human hearing gathered in the 1935–1936 U.S. Public Health Survey. Audiometers used for clinical assessment were required to conform to the ASA standards by ensuring that the output levels matched the reference norm at each frequency. In this way, a "standard" audiogram could be generated that would be instantly meaningful to any other clinic using the same norms. Unfortunately, the data adopted by ASA were influenced by inconsistent data collection methods used in the course of the survey, and by selecting subjects ranging in age from 8 to 74 years only on the basis of their report of "normal" hearing. The normative standards published by the International Standards Organization (ISO) in Europe differed from the ASA standards by an average of about 10 dB; growing concern among investigators about this discrepancy led to the adoption of the ISO norms in 1964. American audiometers were recalibrated to the new standard. This meant that the output reference for "0" on the dial became *lower* by 5 to 15 dB, depending on frequency. Five years later, in 1969, the American National Standards Institute (ANSI; formerly ASA) published yet another set of norms for sound pressure levels as a function of frequency at audiometric 0. Differences in the ISO and ANSI norms differed by 0.2 to 5.5 dB for the earphone in most common clinical usage at the time, the TDH-39. The values for earphone sound pressure level at audiometric 0 under the three standards are shown in Table 2–1. Each value corresponds to output intensity in dB sound pressure level (SPL) re: 20 μbar when the attenuator dial is set to 0 at a particular frequency.

The advantage of having a universally meaningful and comparable audiogram, however, requires that the output standards be maintained; that is, they must be calibrated.

The most important reason why calibration is an absolute requirement for accurate hearing assessment is that, assuming that hearing sensitivity is expressed in dB HL, the numbers on the audiometer's attenuator dial are *completely meaningless* unless they conform to a specified standard for audiometric 0 at each frequency. To illustrate this concept, imagine that a person had a hearing loss at 500 Hz of 50 dB HL using ASA standards. That would correspond to 74.1 dB SPL (24.1 dB SPL for 0 dB HL plus the 50 dB hearing loss). By ISO standards, the same 50 dB on the dial corresponds to 60.1 dB SPL (10.1 for audiometric 0 plus the loss), and by ANSI standards to 61.5 dB SPL. Another way of viewing this situation is to calculate the difference in "sensitivity" expressed in dB HL for a constant loss of 50 dB SPL at 1000 Hz. Using the ASA standard, 50 dB SPL would be about 33 dB HL, whereas it would be 43 dB HL with ISO and ANSI standards. The basic impairment of 50 dB SPL did not change; only the norm to which it was compared changed.

The purpose of the foregoing discussion is not to emphasize differences in organization of various standards, but to show that information about auditory function derived by means of a clinical audiometer is influenced to a significant degree by how closely the output and the reference sound pressure levels are in agreement. As the following discussion illustrates, other acoustic parameters, such as rise time, harmonic distortion, and frequency output, are equally important. Three types of regular equipment checks are recommended: the daily inspection and listening check; the quarterly or monthly calibration; and the annual calibration.

Table 2-1. Values for TDH-39 Earphone Sound Pressure Level Under Three Standard Systems

Frequency	ASA, 1951	ISO, 1964	ANSI, 1969
125	51.8	42.8	45.0
250	39.5	24.5	25.5
500	24.1	10.1	11.5
750		6.5	8.0
1000	17.2	7.2	7.0
1500		8.0	6.5
2000	18.0	9.5	9.0
3000	15.6	7.1	10.0
4000	14.3	8.3	9.5
6000	19.5	10.0	15.5
8000	26.8	15.3	13.0

After Hodgson, W., *Basic Audiologic Evaluation* (1980). Baltimore: Williams and Wilkins, p. 23.

DAILY INSPECTION

At the beginning of each clinical day the audiologist should inspect the equipment and materials to be used for that day's testing. Table 2-2 presents a form useful for completing a daily check. There are three areas that receive attention: (1) area maintenance; (2) the physical appearance of the equipment; and (3) the listening check.

Area Maintenance

Appearances count. The patient's impression of you as a professional and as a representative of your clinic facility begins at first sight, continues to grow with your initial conversation, and is reinforced by the appearance of the testing area. An area with toys strewn across the floor, overflowing wastebaskets, excess papers on desktops, or dusty or soiled equipment does not instill a feeling of confidence on the part of the patient. Cords leading to earphones, patient signal, bone oscillator, and microphones are easily tangled; this condition is unsightly, leads to early cord wear and breakage, and restricts the full extension of the cord between the wall of the testing area and the patient's chair. Because most hearing impaired patients rely to some extent on lipreading, lighting in the counseling or interview room as well as in the testing enclosure should be adequate. Assuring yourself *before* the first patient arrives that

Table 2–2. Daily Equipment Check

DAILY EQUIPMENT CHECK

Audiometer model _____

Date _____

	Initial	Action
I. Area maintenance		
A. Is form supply sufficient?	_____	_____
B. Are tapes in order?	_____	_____
C. Are jacks connected?	_____	_____
D. Are cords untangled?	_____	_____
E. Is test room tidy?	_____	_____
F. Is lighting adequate?	_____	_____
II. Physical inspection of equipment		
A. Are dials loose or out of alignment?	_____	_____
B. Are earphones intact; do they show signs of wear?	_____	_____
C. Do cords show signs of wear?	_____	_____
D. Are instrument panel lights functioning?	_____	_____
E. Does patient response button function?	_____	_____
F. Does visual reinforcement system function?	_____	_____
G. Does tape player function?	_____	_____
III. Listening check		
A. Attenuators (through phones)		
1. Is there smooth intensity change from low to high?	_____	_____
2. Are there audible clicks or roughness?	_____	_____
3. Is background noise present?	_____	_____
B. Signals (*all* output modes)		
1. Is there a clear quality to the pure tones?	_____	_____
2. Is speech (taped and live voice) clear at all intensities?	_____	_____
3. Is masking noise present?	_____	_____
4. Does masking intensity increase smoothly and linearly?	_____	_____
C. Switching		
1. Is the signal equally loud in right and left earphones at same level?	_____	_____
2. Is signal equally loud in right and left speakers?	_____	_____
3. Is there "cross talk" between earphones?	_____	_____
4. Is signal present for each channel?	_____	_____

Action = OK, Repair, Adjust

---

there are enough clinical forms to last through the day and that all tape recorded materials you may need are within reach of the audiometer will avoid having to leave a patient in the middle of an assessment to attend to these tasks.

Physical Inspection of Equipment

Worn or frayed cords constitute electrical hazards and will also result in intermittent or absent signals at the earphone, speakers, or bone oscillator. As discussed in a later section on sources of error in auditory assessment, this may lead to inaccurate conclusions about a patient's response reliability or cooperation. Equipment dials that are loose or out of alignment cannot be considered accurate indicators of output intensity or linearity of attenuation.

Listening Check of Equipment

The listening check of equipment is one of the most important parts of the daily inspection, for the clinician is able to identify problems that could influence patients' test behavior and audiometric results. The discovery of a weak earphone (one that has insufficient output) should come at the beginning of the day, rather than at the end after every patient's test has been invalidated. Patients may respond to audible clicks in the earphone and not to the desired tonal stimuli and thus appear to have "perfect" hearing at all frequencies. Conversely, background noise such as buzzing, humming, or scratchiness on the channel may mask the signal at low intensities, leading to artificially elevated threshold estimates.

There should be no obvious distortion of pure tones or speech stimuli, and all signals should sound the same through each earphone and when generated by each channel. There should never be "cross-talk" in the earphones (i.e., having a signal present in each phone when it should be limited to only one).

Many of these problems can arise either from within the electronic circuitry of the audiometer or from a transducer (earphone, speaker, bone oscillator). Assume, for example, that the right earphone has been noted to have very weak output. Is the problem in the earphone or in the audiometer? One easy way to check is to plug the right earphone plug into the left phone jack on the audiometer. If the earphone is at fault, the signal will be weak when the signal is put out to the left phone; if the audiometer is at fault, the signal will be nor l under the same circumstance. Problems such as these most (en result from faulty earphones that have been damaged by dropping or hitting them or by directing inappropriately high intensities through them. For this reason, every clinic should be equipped with at least one spare set of earphones and a bone oscillator for each audiometer. If an earphone problem is identified, then, testing can continue. If the problem appears to lie within the audiometer, it is best not to use that equipment until it has been inspected and any necessary repairs have been made.

Equipment used for immittance audiometry should also be inspected carefully. There should be an adequate supply of clean, dry probe tips, and specula for an otoscope. Table 2–3 presents a check list that can be used to conduct a daily check on an immittance bridge.

As a final word, it is important to emphasize that a listening check is just a *check* and should not be equated to or considered a substitute for a formal electroacoustic calibration for any piece of equipment.

MONTHLY OR QUARTERLY CHECKS

On the topic of electroacoustic calibration procedures, the reader is referred to Wilber (1985). There is, to this author's knowledge and opinion, no more complete, easily read, and informative discussion of that subject available today.

There is no general agreement as to whether electroacoustic calibration checks should take place monthly, quarterly, or only annually. My personal opinion is that equipment should be checked more frequently than once a year, especially if it is older than 1 or 2 years. However, new equipment is no guarantee that calibration is perfect, and the apparatus should be checked as soon as it is unpacked and installed in the testing area.

Hodgson (1980) recommends that quarterly calibrations include the following areas: sound pressure level output from both earphones, attenuator linearity, and bone conduction oscillator output and function. Annual calibrations would repeat those measurements and add study of frequency output, signal rise-fall time, and quantification of harmonic distortion. These procedures constitute the minimum areas for electroacoustic calibration; Wilber (1985) also includes discussion of procedures for determining SPL of masking noises and speech signals; behavioral and electroacoustic methods of checking loudspeaker and bone conduction oscillator output; checking of special test equipment; and determining whether the sound attenuating properties of the test enclosure are in accordance with ANSI standards.

After the SPL output of the equipment transducers has been measured, the values should be compared to the standards for audiometric 0 published by the American National Standards Institute (ANSI S3.6-1969 [R1973]). The SPL output should be within ±3 dB

Table 2-3. Immittance Bridge Check

IMMITTANCE BRIDGE CHECK

Equipment model _____

Date _____

Procedure	Initial	Action
1. From the manometer, determine air pressure in mm H_2O at +200, 0, and −200 mm. Variations >25 mm require adjustment.	_____	_____
2. Is the pressure held with no leaks?	_____	_____
3. Is probe tone present and at appropriate intensity?	_____	_____
4. Calibrate compliance for 0.2 and 4.0 (or 5.0) cc cavity.	_____	_____
5. Are pure tones present at all frequencies for both ipsilateral and contralateral activation?	_____	_____
6. Does pure tone attenuator change smoothly and linearly?	_____	_____
7. Is there any distortion or warble in the pure tone stimuli?	_____	_____

Action = OK, Adjust, Repair

---

of the standard for the frequencies 500 to 4000 Hz and within ±5 dB at other frequencies. If the discrepancy between reference and output is unacceptably large at any frequency, a *correction sheet* must be posted adjacent to the audiometer. These correction values are used by the clinician when recording measured thresholds. Corrections are rounded off to the nearest 5 dB. Thus, a deviation of 7 dB from the norm would result in a 10 dB correction being applied. An example of such a correction sheet is shown in Table 2-4.

If corrections of 15 dB at any frequency or 10 dB at three or more frequencies are posted, the equipment should be inspected and repaired if necessary by qualified technical personnel. The development and increasing prevalence of audiometers with accessible "trim pots" now makes on-site audiometer correction possible. As these newer instruments replace their predecessors, the necessity to post correction sheets will be gradually eliminated.

The validity and accuracy of auditory assessment procedures requires test equipment that is properly calibrated and maintained.

Table 2–4.   Correction Sheet for Audiometer

Transducer	Frequency, Hz									
	125	250	500	1000	1500	2000	3000	4000	6000	8000
Right										
Left										
Bone										

+ dB = Audiometer strong, make threshold *higher*
− dB = Audiometer weak, make threshold *lower*

It is the responsibility of the audiologist to see that calibration and maintenance are up to date. Should the audiologist ever be required to testify about his or her test results in a legal action, one of the first questions asked will concern the calibration status at the time of the questioned evaluation. Failure to demonstrate correct calibration could lead to accusations of professional negligence in the worst case and to invalidation of the testimony in the best. For these reasons, if a patient's auditory status is known to be at issue in a litigation process, many audiologists will take care to carry out complete electroacoustic calibration checks with the equipment *on the day* that the patient is to be tested. By so doing, one important source of potential error in the evaluation process will be eliminated or at least identified and corrected for.

STUDY QUESTIONS

1. What does audiometric zero mean?
2. How do different norms influence calculation of degree of hearing loss?
3. What would be the effect on threshold measurements of an audiometer with output 10 dB *higher* than the norm? 10 dB *lower* than the norm?
4. Why should a listening check be performed on a daily basis?

Chapter 3

Preliminary Procedures

THE CASE HISTORY

The late Dr. Philip Rosenberg made an important point when he described the case history as "the first test" in the auditory assessment (1978). Experienced clinicians know that the time they spend interviewing the patient prior to beginning formal test procedures can help to establish preliminary hypotheses about the nature of a patient's complaint. The same observations or impressions can be used later as a form of cross-check against the test results. The importance of this initial contact cannot be overemphasized; no matter how busy the testing situation or whether a medical history is already available, the few minutes of interaction with the patient before beginning test procedures should not be relinquished.

The goals of a case history taken for medical purposes and one taken for auditory assessment are both similar and different. In the medical situation, the information is needed to establish a physical diagnosis, a function which is the exclusive privilege of the physician. The specific aim is to determine the cause of a hearing impairment and thus to select the appropriate medical or surgical treatment. Note that the medical model involves establishing the nature of a disease or pathological condition, a process for which the physician has become qualified through medical education. However, Miller (1985) quite appropriately notes that diagnosis can also be viewed as an orderly process of systematic and scientific observations leading to an understanding of the nature of something. Within this viewpoint, it is not inappropriate for an audiologist to "diagnose" a conductive or sensorineural auditory dysfunction, which the physician's diagnosis might demonstrate to be due to otosclerosis or Meniere's disease. The purpose of the history in auditory assessment is also to lead to the proper management plan—medical referral, hearing aid fitting, counseling, and so forth—and to reconcile the patient's auditory complaint with the results of the evaluation. Here the extent of the history will vary with the goals of the evaluation. If it is primarily diagnostic, more emphasis will be given to physical symptoms and to the natural history, or course, of the auditory problem. These details are then used to support the impression of a site of disorder suggested by the test battery. For example, when the evaluation is focused on disability rating, diagnostic information will be of secondary concern to information about the social communicative effects of the disorder.

The initial contact consists of observation of the patient. Taking note of certain details such as those described in the following paragraphs will remind you of particular areas of the case history that may need more complete questioning; they can also alert you to the possibility of a central nervous system (CNS) disorder as a potential contributor to auditory dysfunction.

Gender and Apparent Age

Males of all ages are more likely to have had some history of recreational or occupational noise exposure, and of course older persons often have some degree of age-related hearing impairment.

Presence of Hearing Aids

A person wearing hearing aids will almost certainly have been through one or more hearing evaluations in the past; knowledge of these results will help establish whether a hearing impairment is stable, fluctuating, or progressive and whether the patient has been able to benefit from amplification.

Facial or Cranial Asymmetry or Malformation

Craniofacial anomalies are often associated with anomalies in the middle or inner ear, or in both. Facial paralysis or weakness may signal retrocochlear disorder. Look at the patient's face and eyes while introducing yourself. A *natural* white forelock and irises of different colors are signs of Waardenburg's syndrome, in which sensorineural hearing impairment is prevalent. Certain abnormalities of the cornea can be found in patients with congenital syphilis, which can mimic the symptoms of Meniere's disease. Note any repetitive, involuntary eye movements from side to side or up and down *(nystagmus)* that seem to have a slow deviation from the midline and a faster return to the midline. Nystagmus is normal under certain circumstances, such as counting the cars on a moving freight train or following a series of moving stripes. Under most other circumstances, it is considered a sign of peripheral or central vestibular disorder. Nystagmus is usually observable only with eyes closed in peripheral disturbances; its presence with eyes open and visual fixation is considered suggestive of a central origin. Patients with congenital visual disturbances or pigmentation defects, however, often have nystagmus without vestibular disorders.

Evidence of Physical Disability or Neuromuscular Disorder

Neuromuscular disorders such as multiple sclerosis, cerebral palsy, and myasthenia gravis often are associated with particular auditory abnormalities. When hand and arm weakness is present, modifications in the way the patient is instructed to respond during the test will be necessary.

Apparent Ability to Attend to Speech Informally

By calling the patient's name and then introducing yourself at a normal conversational intensity, you can quickly estimate the extent to which hearing might be impaired for ordinary speech. At this time it is also important to observe whether the patient is making good eye contact, avoiding eye contact, or watching your lips. Individuals with nonorganic types of impairment often exaggerate their problem by failing to respond to several repetitions of their name or by calling your attention to the fact that they have to lipread. By contrast, individuals with valid organic impairment have usually developed compensatory strategies for dealing with their impairment and may appear to function quite well.

The trip between waiting room and testing area provides another opportunity for observation. Allowing the patient to precede you slightly permits assessment of his or her balance and walking pattern. A broad-based, staggering, or otherwise unsteady walk (ataxia) suggests some CNS disorder, especially one affecting the cerebellum. Patients who consistently deviate to the right or left while attempting to walk a straight line may have a disorder affecting the vestibular apparatus. At this time you can also ask a few questions (e.g., "Did you have trouble parking?" "Have you lived in this city long?") at a soft-to-normal vocal intensity to continue an informal assessment of hearing for speech when visual cues necessary for lipreading are not available.

Once the patient is seated comfortably, the case history can be started. Ideally, the interview room will have an overhead light source; if not, the patient should be seated in such a way that the light is *behind* the patient's head, thus illuminating the clinician's face and facilitating lipreading. Some clinics routinely take a history "from scratch," that is, an in-depth interview covering all areas without prior information from the patient or referral source. Others find it more convenient to ask the patient to complete a pre-printed history form before the evaluation and mail it back to the clinic, where the clinician can study it and plan an interview strategy. This method also has the advantage of allowing the patient to think about and to respond to questions in a more leisurely and relaxed way. The subsequent interview then is used to explore in greater depth those areas in which some abnormality or risk factor has been noted on the questionnaire. An example of such a form is provided at the end of this chapter.

A very useful technique for beginning an interview is to ask the patient what has brought him or her to your facility for assessment. Listening "between the lines" alerts you to social factors (for example, "My wife says I need a hearing aid") that may subtly influence a patient's motivation and level of cooperation.

The case history, whether obtained verbally or from a form, should include information in the following areas.

Identifying Information

This section is used for record-keeping and can also be used for data retrieval. It should include the patient's name, mailing address, telephone number, date of birth, referral source, evaluation date, and the clinician's name.

Presenting Complaint

It is helpful in this section to write the patient's description of the problem in his or her exact words, if possible. Usually patients will give you all the information you require with little prompting. Basically, you will wish to know whether *the patient* (not spouse or children or employer) feels that he or she has a hearing impairment; which ear is affected; how long the problem has been noticeable; whether it had a sudden or gradual onset; whether it is stable or fluctuating; and whether he or she has ever had a similar problem. If the hearing impairment had a sudden onset, the patient will usually be able to relate its onset to a specific time or event (e.g., being around an explosion or having a flu-like illness). If it has been more gradual, the clinician can sometimes help the patient date the loss by asking him or her to relate its onset or presence to significant life events—before or after retirement, birth of last child, move to present home, and so forth.

Accompanying Symptoms

Because of the close proximity of auditory structures to other cranial vessels, nerves, and organs, hearing impairment is often accompanied by other nonauditory symptoms; sometimes these other symptoms constitute the major concern to the patient and may even be stated as the chief complaint. One of the most common auditory problems is *tinnitus:* subjectively perceived noises usually described as ringing, roaring, buzzing, hissing, chirping, throbbing, humming, or clicking sounds in one or both ears. It is important to obtain as clear a description of the tinnitus as possible, as well as its relationship to other auditory or vestibular symptoms. What does the tinnitus sound like? Is it present constantly or intermittently? In one or both ears? Does it change its quality (i.e., become louder or change pitch from time to time)? When did the tinnitus start relative to the onset of the hearing impairment? Can the patient make the tinnitus appear or disappear by any voluntary action, such as changing head or body position? Is it more noticeable at certain times of day?

The answers to these questions can help in some cases to identify the source of the tinnitus. High-pitched tinnitus usually appears with cochlear involvement, whereas low-pitched roaring is seen most often with middle ear or occasionally retrocochlear disorders. A pulsatile tinnitus may signal the presence of a vascular abnormality in the middle ear (glomus jugulare). Intermittent clicking sounds have been reported with palatal myoclonus (a kind of tic of the soft palate) and with tonic contraction of the middle ear muscles. Sometimes these sounds are not purely subjective but can be heard by another person, usually with a stethoscope. A rhythmic rushing tinnitus ("like wind blowing") is often experienced by individuals with a patulous or abnormally open eustachian tube; it is indeed the sound of "wind"—the patient's own—that he or she hears during the respiratory cycle. This form of tinnitus is sometimes found among patients who have lost a great deal of weight; it may be absent for a short while after arising in the morning, when local nasopharyngeal congestion around the eustachian tube makes the effect less noticeable. Other forms of head noises (e.g., voices or music) suggest auditory hallucinations and the patient should be referred to a physician.

Another common symptom that may appear with auditory dysfunction is *vertigo* or other forms of "dizziness" and dysequilibrium. Classic vertigo is always characterized by a rotary component—a sensation of spinning. If the patient feels as if he or she is spinning, either around and around or head over heels, the sensation is described as *subjective vertigo.* If, on the other hand, he perceives himself to be stationary while the room or environment spins, it is called *objective vertigo.* Both subjective and objective forms of vertigo are produced by peripheral vestibular disturbances and are largely related to whether a patient has his or her eyes open or closed. However, true vertigo is rarely produced by the more serious central conditions, often appearing as vague types of dysequilibrium. If a patient reports "dizziness" in a case history he or she should be carefully questioned to determine whether this represents "true" vertigo. Although vertigo is usually accompanied by nystagmus, the nystagmus may not be obvious when the patient's eyes are open.

Many other forms of dysequilibrium exist, some more benign than others. When questioned, patients often report lightheadedness, faintness, a feeling of disorientation in space or of being "off balance." One patient with retrocochlear dysfunction struggled for words to describe her feeling, then said, "It's like trying to walk on Jello!" Other patients with similar disorders have compared their dysequilibrium to learning to walk on a ship at sea. Not unexpectedly, nausea (a term derived from the Greek word for sea!) and vomiting are often side effects of vertigo and other forms of dysequilibrium produced when the peripheral and central vestibular systems are affected.

Some accompanying symptoms are referred directly to the ears. Two common symptoms are aural *fullness* and *pain.* Fullness may be described as feeling as if the ear were stopped up or as if there were water in the ear. Pain may be referred to the ear canal, to the mastoid area, to deep within the ear, or to the scalp area surrounding the pinna. Ear pain that is most noticeable while eating or chewing may be produced by temporomandibular joint (TMJ) dysfunction, a condition known to produce tinnitus and certain kinds of dysequilibrium as well (Arlen, 1977).

During this part of the history, the patient should also be questioned about any feelings of facial *numbness* or reduced sensation, *tingling*, or *weakness* and the relationship of these symptoms in time to the onset of auditory symptoms. Positive answers to these questions or to questions about any difficulty in articulation, chewing, swallowing, or word-finding indicate that the clinician should be alert to signs of retrocochlear dysfunction during the subsequent evaluation. Symptoms of these kinds also mean that, if not already under medical supervision, the patient should be referred to a physician without delay.

Communication History

This part of the history is devoted to obtaining some preliminary information about the ways and situations in which an auditory disorder affects social communication efficiency. The most prevalent complaint among individuals with sensorineural hearing impairment is marked difficulty in understanding speech when there is noise in the background. Equally common is the complaint, "I can hear people talking, but I can't understand what they're saying" or "[Speech] is loud enough but not clear enough." These complaints are very uncommon among individuals with conductive hearing impairment, because their problem is a simple one of attenuation—if the speech is made loud enough, they can hear normally.

A very important goal of the communication history is to determine situations in which the patient finds the hearing impairment to be a handicap, as well as his or her psychological attitude toward the impairment. A person who leads a quiet, secluded life might find the same hearing impairment to be less of a communication handicap than would a busy executive; on the other hand, he or she may find inability to enjoy music or to hear bird songs psychologically devastating. This information will also be extremely useful for counseling and rehabilitative purposes.

Throughout the interview the clinician should observe the patient's receptive and expressive communicative ability. Does the patient rely to a large extent on lipreading for communication? Does he or she respond appropriately to questions or is repetition consistently required? Is the patient's voice excessively loud or soft?

(Patients with bilateral cochlear disorders often speak very loudly in an effort to maintain auditory feedback for monitoring speech output. Those with middle ear disorders, on the other hand, may speak softly because competing environmental noises are attenuated by the hearing impairment, but their own speech production is monitored effectively by the mechanism of bone conduction.) Does the patient exhibit consistent errors of articulation? Are there inappropriate vocal pitch patterns? (These characteristics suggest fairly severe bilateral sensorineural hearing loss of long duration.) If the patient is wearing a hearing aid, does it generate feedback (a high-pitched squeal) or require constant adjustment?

Family History

In many instances, the exact origin of hearing impairment, especially sensorineural impairment, cannot be identified; in others, a clear pattern of genetic transmission or familial tendency can be identified. If there is such a pattern, referral for genetic counseling or study may be indicated; this would have the additional benefit of alerting the family to other members who might be affected. If the patient indicates that another family member is or was hearing impaired, he or she should be questioned as to which member, when the loss occurred, what kind of impairment it was, whether it became progressively worse, and what was done about it. Patients with family histories of hearing impairment should be reevaluated annually to assess the stability of the impairment and to update recommendations for its management. The children of hearing impaired adults should be evaluated as well if there is any indication of a familial pattern and if the parent's hearing impairment appears to be progressive.

Noise Exposure History

One of the most prevalent sources of hearing impairment today is traumatic noise exposure. With modern (and powerful) sound generating equipment a part of nearly every child's experience, it is no longer necessary to be old enough for military experience, full time employment, or use of firearms to acquire a noise-induced hearing loss; in our own clinic, we have tested children 8 to 10 years old who have substantial hearing impairment related to consistent use of earphones on portable tape players. A recent study reported that such devices are capable of maximum sound output of up to 120 dB SPL! Other possible contemporary sources of traumatic noise include motorcycles, snowmobiles, all-terrain cycles, and power tools. The history of noise exposure should include a description of the type of noise, the average duration of exposure, how long the patient has had that type of exposure, whether ear protection is worn, and whether the patient notices changes in auditory status (e.g., hearing loss, tinnitus, aural fullness) after the noise exposure.

General Medical History

This section can be divided into several subsections: First, the patient's general health at the present time; second, the record of past illnesses and their treatment; third, the specific otologic history; and fourth, medications currently used by the patient.

In addition to eliciting a statement from the patient about general health (whether it is "excellent," "good," "fair," or "poor"), the clinician should ask specifically about conditions that may be directly related to the patient's auditory status, such as heart disease (including high blood pressure) or diseases of the kidneys, liver, or nervous system, and how they are being treated. All patients should be asked whether they have diabetes or cardiovascular disease, with the realization that obese patients are particularly at risk for these conditions, which are associated with sensorineural hearing loss.

Past illnesses such as meningitis, measles, mumps, or whooping cough may have contributed to a hearing loss. The history of certain other diseases may be important because they are usually treated with drugs known to be toxic to the ear: tuberculosis may have been treated with streptomycin, malaria with quinine, certain severe infections with kanamycin or gentamycin, rheumatoid arthritis with large doses of aspirin, and "valley fever" (coccidioidomycosis) with amphotericin B.

Any type of middle ear infection, of course, may have been responsible for a conductive hearing impairment, and middle ear surgery may leave residual hearing losses. This section of the history should include specific information about past or present otologic management, the name of the otologist, conditions for which the patient is undergoing treatment, and types and dates (if possible) of surgery on the ear.

Blows to the head resulting in concussion or skull fracture can cause either conductive or sensorineural hearing impairment. Finally, the patient should be asked about medications—both prescription and over-the-counter—that he or she currently uses. Optimally, the reason for the drug and its dosage will be recorded. It is not uncommon for patients with vague dysequilibrium or tinnitus to provide a list of 10 or more medications which they take daily! The use of oral contraceptives should be determined, because they have been associated (in a small percentage of users) with the formation of blood clots that could be related to peripheral or central auditory dysfunction.

Social History

This is a very brief section that covers the patient's occupation, chief recreational interests, and use of tobacco and alcohol. This information yields insight into factors that could have caused or worsened a hearing impairment and helps provide a framework for designing a personal hearing conservation program. Recent research has established that acoustic reflex thresholds are raised by alcohol (Bauch and Robinette, 1978; Borg and Møller, 1968).

Previous Audiologic Management

In this section you will inquire if the patient has had previous hearing evaluations and if he or she knows what the results were. At this point, eager patients will sometimes turn over a sheaf of previous audiograms; these will be useful for comparison with the results of the present evaluation to determine the stability of the loss. If the patient is new to you, it is probably better to defer study of the other audiograms until you have completed your own assessment, objectively and free from the influence of other results.

Certainly, the history of previous hearing aid experience is of interest. This history should include what kind(s) of amplification systems were used, which ear was fit, and, importantly, the patient's satisfaction with amplification. It is also important to be aware of any aural habilitation or rehabilitation that has been implemented and the patient's opinion of the effectiveness of the programs. Such information allows the clinician to design a management plan that may sidestep factors that have been a barrier to effective communication in the past.

At the beginning of the interview the patient was asked to explain what he or she perceived to be the chief problem. At the end of the interview it is useful to give him or her the same sort of opportunity by asking, "Is there anything else that *you* feel is important for me to know about your problem that we haven't discussed?" Some patients are quite talkative and will, with very little encouragement, volunteer all the information needed for a complete history—and often much more. Other patients are more reticent, either by nature or out of anxiety, and will limit their responses to specific questions. If the question is not asked, the information is not forthcoming.

Before testing commences, the patient should be asked to identify the professionals or facilities to which he or she would like to have the reports of the evaluation sent. It is necessary for the patient to sign a release of information form allowing your clinic to send this confidential information *only* to those places he or she designates. Similarly, if you wish to include other medical records of the patient's in your chart, he or she must sign a release permitting the other facility to release those records directly to yours.

The patient and the clinician should each enter the testing situation with some expectations in mind. The patient has a general idea of what the test will involve and how long it will take. The clinician carries some preliminary hypotheses about the likelihood of auditory disorder, its possible site, and its effect on communication, developed by careful observation of the patient and by attention to the details of the history. The evaluation is used to accept, modify, or reject these hypotheses by continued observation of the patient during application of a battery of tests selected to be appropriate for the goals of the evaluation. Table 3–1 shows a sample form for history taking.

STUDY QUESTIONS

1. What is tinnitus?
2. Distinguish between vertigo and dysequilibrium.
3. How is the case history used to develop some hypotheses about the nature of an auditory problem?

Table 3–1.   Form for Taking the Case History

ADULT CASE HISTORY

Name _____ Sex _____ Birthdate _____

Address _____ Phone _____

Occupation (now) _____ (formerly) _____

Referred by _____ File # _____

I. Subjective: Hearing History

A.   Do you have any problem hearing? ☐ Yes   ☐ No
Which ear? ☐ Right ☐ Left ☐ Both
When did you first notice it? _____
Has the hearing loss been: ☐ Gradual ☐ Sudden ☐ Fluctuating

B.   Have you ever had a hearing test? ☐ Yes ☐ No
Where _____
When? _____
Results (if known) _____

C.   Do you wear a hearing aid? ☐ Yes ☐ No
How long have you worn it? _____
Are you satisfied with it? _____

D.   If no, have you ever thought about using a hearing aid? ☐ Yes ☐ No

E.   Do you have trouble hearing in any of these situations?

On the telephone	Always	Sometimes	Never
With background noise	Always	Sometimes	Never
Watching television	Always	Sometimes	Never
Children talking	Always	Sometimes	Never
Women talking	Always	Sometimes	Never
Men talking	Always	Sometimes	Never
In movies	Always	Sometimes	Never
In concerts	Always	Sometimes	Never
At parties	Always	Sometimes	Never
At church	Always	Sometimes	Never

F.   Do you hear any noises in your ears? ☐ Yes ☐ No

Describe: ☐ Ringing ☐ Roaring ☐ Buzzing ☐ Chirping ☐ Pulsing ☐ Hissing
☐ Humming ☐ Other _____

These noises are in ☐ Right ear ☐ Left ear ☐ Both ears
The noises are present ☐ Always ☐ Often ☐ Sometimes
When did you start having the noises? _____

G.   Have you had any dizziness? ☐ Yes ☐ No
Which of the following describes your dizziness?
☐ The room seems like it's spinning and I'm still
☐ I feel like I'm spinning and the room is still
☐ I feel lightheaded
☐ I feel like I'm going to fall down
☐ I feel sick to my stomach

(continued on next page)

Table 3–1 (*continued*).

    ☐ I feel off-balance in space
    ☐ Other (describe) _____
    ☐ When did you start feeling dizzy? _____
    Is your dizziness caused by any particular body movement? ☐ Yes ☐ No
    What movement? _____
    The dizziness is present ☐ Always ☐ Often ☐ Sometimes

H.   Do you have a feeling of fullness or pain in your ears? ☐ Yes ☐ No
    That feeling is present ☐ Always ☐ Often ☐ Sometimes
    The feeling is present in ☐ Right ear ☐ Left ear ☐ Both
    When did you start having that feeling? _____

II. Otologic History

A.   Have you had repeated ear infections? ☐ Yes ☐ No
    Which ear? ☐ Right ☐ Left ☐ Both ☐ Can't remember

B.   Are you presently being treated by an ear specialist? ☐ Yes ☐ No
    For what reason? _____
    Physician's name _____

C.   Have you ever had surgery on your ears? ☐ Yes ☐ No
    Type of surgery _____
    Date of surgery _____

D.   Have you ever been exposed to loud noises? ☐ Yes ☐ No
    Please indicate the types of noise:

    ☐ Gunfire   ☐ Motorcycles
    ☐ Explosions   ☐ Power lawn mowers
    ☐ Factory noise   ☐ Aircraft
    ☐ Power tools   ☐ Loud music
    ☐ Heavy equipment   ☐ Military tanks
    ☐ Other types _____
    Do you think that noise has affected your hearing? ☐ Yes ☐ No

III. Family History

Has any blood relative that you know of had a hearing loss? ☐ Yes ☐ No
What was the cause of the hearing loss? _____
How was the(se) person(s) related to you?

☐ Father   ☐ Grandfather
☐ Mother   ☐ Aunt
☐ Sister   ☐ Uncle
☐ Brother   ☐ Cousin
☐ Grandmother   ☐ Child

IV. General Medical History

A.   Health at present can best be described as _____

B.   Do you have diabetes? ☐ Yes ☐ No
    Age at onset _____
    Treatment (diet, drugs, etc.) _____

(continued on next page)

Table 3–1 (*continued*).

C.   Do you have high blood pressure? ☐ Yes ☐ No
Approximate age at onset _____
Treatment _____

D.   Do you have heart or kidney disease? ☐ Yes ☐ No
Type and age of onset _____
Treatment _____

E.   Please indicate which of the following diseases you have had. State approximate age or date of onset.

_____ Measles	_____ Rheumatic fever	_____ Malaria
_____ Mumps	_____ Scarlet fever	_____ TB
_____ Chickenpox	_____ Diphtheria	_____ Cancer
_____ Polio	_____ Meningitis	_____ Venereal disease
_____ Pneumonia	_____ Severe burns	_____ Epilepsy
_____ Jaundice	_____ Valley fever	_____ Other

F.   Do you take any medication regularly? ☐ Yes ☐ No
Type and dosage _____

G.   Do you smoke cigarettes or cigars? ☐ Yes ☐ No
How much do you smoke per day (packs)? _____
How long have you been smoking (years)? _____

H.   Do you drink alcohol: ☐ Regularly ☐ Socially ☐ Never

V. Communication History

A.   Does your hearing loss interfere with communication? ☐ Yes ☐ No

B.   Have you been enrolled in an aural rehabilitation program? ☐ Yes ☐ No
Did it seem to help you? ☐ Yes ☐ No

C.   Has your hearing problem affected your relationships with family or friends?
☐ Yes ☐ No

D.   Are you able to use lipreading efficiently? ☐ Yes ☐ No

To whom should we send a report of this evaluation?
Name _____
Address _____
_____

Chapter 4

Principles and Measurement of Acoustic Impedance

This chapter represents something of a departure from the clinical tone established in the preceding chapters and in those to follow. The discussion is intended to provide a foundation for understanding and interpreting the results of impedance measures.

The introduction of techniques to measure acoustic impedance and admittance had the most profound influence on clinical hearing assessment since the development of the electric audiometer. These techniques provided a relatively inexpensive, easily applied, and noninvasive method for evaluating middle ear integrity and for differentiating among types of otologic abnormalities. A further advantage was that voluntary responses from the subject were not required. Later work demonstrated the clinical utility of acoustic reflex measurement in distinguishing between cochlear and retrocochlear sites of auditory dysfunction. Next came the application of these tests to mass auditory screening in schools. They proved to be a more sensitive tool than pure tone screening for identifying middle ear dysfunction, which is the most common cause of acquired hearing impairment in children. Evidence of the versatility of acoustic impedance and admittance measurements is found in their application to the assessment of neuromuscular disorders such as myasthenia gravis and multiple sclerosis, prediction of sensori-neural impairment, location of facial nerve dysfunction, and as an aid to determining amplification settings for hearing aids. Perhaps the most significant contribution of "impedance audiometry" has been as the cornerstone of the cross-check principle. For example, the results can be used to verify and support behavioral evidence of conductive hearing impairment, retrocochlear eighth nerve disor-der, and nonorganic hearing loss.

It is an interesting paradox that this very important tool is, unlike pure tone audiometry and speech audiometry, based on *indi-rect* measurement. The method relies not on the usual direct stimulus-response observations, but on a series of inferences and on a model of the way in which sound transmission is affected by cer-tain variables of the transmitting system. For example, tympano-metry is based on the effects of pressure gradients across the tympanic membrane and on the relationship between volume and sound pressure level. Understanding acoustic reflex dynamics requires a knowledge of middle ear mechanics, the effects of stiff-ness, mass, and resistance on the transmission of sounds of various frequencies, and principles of neural reflex arcs.

In the clinical application of impedance measures, we do not measure the integrity of the middle ear structures *directly*, only the efficiency with which a low frequency tone is transmitted. We do not measure the action of the stapedius muscle *directly*, only its effect on the acoustic impedance or admittance of the ear. Thus, an understanding of the principles and deductive logic underlying the measurement of acoustic impedance and admittance is critical if test results are to be understood and interpreted correctly.

WHAT IS IMPEDANCE?

First, a definition: "Impedance is the total opposition offered by a system to the flow of energy" (Lilly, 1973, p. 353).

That concept can be considered in more familiar terms: the "flow of energy" can be represented by the velocity of some moving object, such as your arm. Now imagine that you want to compare the impedance of two "systems," represented by a volume of water and a volume of air. You will find that it is more difficult to move your arm in the water than it is in the air: the water offers more opposition to the flow of energy and thus is said to have a higher impedance (Z). To move your arm equally fast in both media, you would have to use more force when your arm was in water. Therefore, impedance can be described by the ratio of achieved velocity (V) to applied force (F). Thus,

$$\text{Impedance} = \text{Force} / \text{Velocity}$$
$$Z = F/V$$

If a force of 10 produced a velocity of 2 in one system and 40 in another, the first system would be said to have a higher impedance than the second: $Z = 10/2 = 5$, versus $Z = 10/40 = 0.25$. Similarly, it would take less force to achieve a criterion velocity of 10 in the lower impedance system:

$$5 = F/10 \qquad \text{versus} \qquad 0.25 = F/10$$
$$F = 50 \qquad\qquad\qquad\qquad F = 2.5$$

The foregoing greatly simplified account of impedance supposes a constant force over some unit of time and is used to describe mechanical impedance. We are interested in acoustic impedance, however, or the opposition offered by a system to an oscillating force that we define as sound.

POWER, PRESSURE, AND VOLUME

Acoustic impedance is measured clinically by determining the sound pressure level of a constant frequency and intensity tone in an enclosed volume of air under various conditions. Therefore, the equation describing mechanical impedance is modified slightly to describe acoustic impedance:

$$\text{Acoustic impedance} = \text{Pressure} / \text{Volume velocity}$$
$$Z_A = P/V_U$$

An understanding of the ways in which power, pressure, and volume covary, therefore, is basic to an understanding of the clinical technique; more importantly, it is essential to interpreting results of clinical impedance measurements. The following discussion is patterned after Newman and Fanger's (1973) excellent tutorial on the topic.

Consider an experimental condition like that shown in Figure 4–1. There are two hard-walled cavities (A and B), a sound source (C) that can deliver a tone into the cavities, and a microphone (D) that is led into a sound level meter (E). When sound is delivered into the cavities with a given force, the sound pressure level in the cavity is an indication of the force per unit area; that is, how much force is applied to all the surfaces of the cavity. Sound pressure level

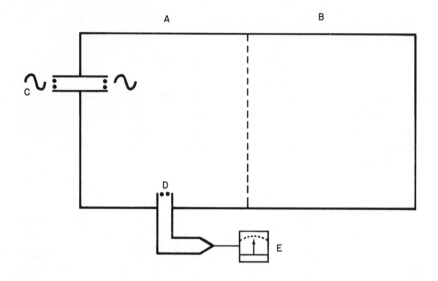

Figure 4–1. Schematic diagram of a system designed to measure sound pressure level in a closed cavity. A sound of a constant intensity is directed into a cavity of a known volume. A microphone in the floor of the cavity collects the sound and directs it to a sound level meter that displays the sound pressure level on a meter.

can be increased in two ways. First, the power at the sound source can be increased, which will increase the force per unit area, because the volume of the cavity has remained constant. A given amount of sound energy delivered into a given volume produces a given pressure; if the energy is changed, the pressure is changed, provided that the volume remains constant. Thus, the second way of increasing the sound pressure level is to decrease the volume, as in Figure 4–2, where cavity B has been detached. If the source power is held constant, sound pressure level again rises, because there is a smaller area over which the force can be distributed. This situation can be compared to turning your radio on to maximum and listening to it first in an auditorium, then in your living room, then in a closet, and finally through earphones. The power at the source does not increase, but the force per unit area does, in a most dramatic way!

RESISTANCE, STIFFNESS, AND MASS

The following sections discuss three properties of matter that can offer opposition to the flow of energy. Although these three proper-

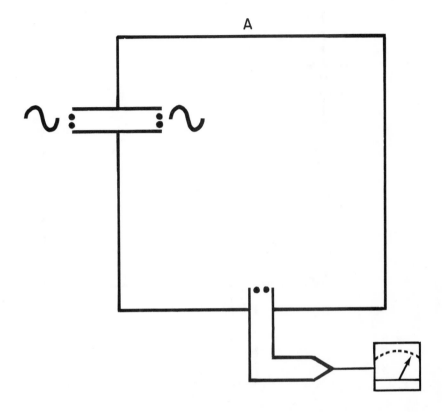

Figure 4-2. Removal of cavity B results in increased sound pressure level because the force per unit area has increased, even though the intensity of the tone at its source is held constant.

ties usually act in combination, their effects will be first considered individually. Keep in mind that, unlike mechanical impedance, which opposes a constant force in one direction, acoustic impedance must account for a time-varying opposition to a "positive" force (condensation) as well as to a "negative" force (rarefaction) and for all points between those extremes.

Resistance

Cavity A of Figure 4-1 will be modified as shown in Figure 4-3: one wall has been replaced with a plate that has several small holes drilled into it. Now, when sound of constant intensity and frequency is directed into the box, the microphone will record lower sound pressure than when the wall was solid. Because both the cavity

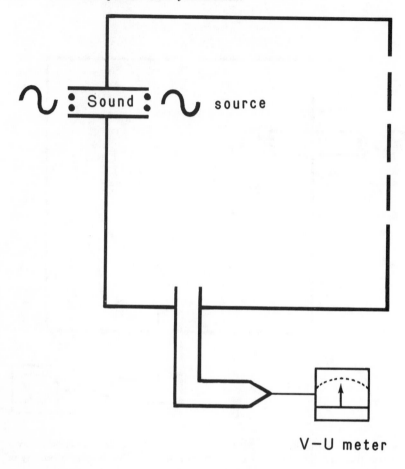

Figure 4–3. When sound is introduced into a cavity that is *not* closed but allows some sound energy to "escape" through the perforated end plate, the SPL is lower than would be predicted on the basis of the volume of the cavity.

volume and the power of the sound source have remained constant, it appears that some of the pressure has been relieved through the perforations. At the same time, however, friction has been created by the air molecules colliding with one another and with the edges of the perforations as they escape from the cavity. Thus, some of the sound energy that was being transmitted has been converted into heat, with a net loss of energy. The processes that permit such losses are called resistance and are common to most situations in which one kind of energy is transformed into another. The middle ear accounts for two such energy transformations: molecular energy is converted to mechanical energy at the tympanic membrane, and mechanical energy is transformed into hydraulic energy at the interface of the stapes footplate and the vestibular fluids. The major sources of resistance in the middle ear, then, are at those two sites, with some slight contributions from the suspensory ligaments of the ossicles.

In the foregoing example pressure and energy flow covary in a predictable way. When pressure at the sound source is maximum, the flow of energy—both within and outside of the cavity—is also at a maximum. Similarly, when pressure is at a minimum, energy flow is at a minimum as well. Therefore, the two factors, pressure and flow, are completely in phase with one another. This relationship is shown in Figure 4–4.

Stiffness ($-X_C$)

In a hard-walled cavity such as those in the previous two examples, the stiffness of the walls has been uniform. To study the effect of stiffness on sound pressure and energy flow, the perforated end

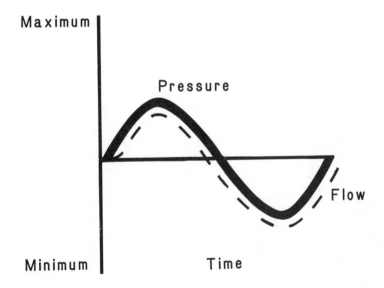

Figure 4–4. In a system characterized by resistance only, such as that shown in Figure 4–3, sound pressure (solid line) and flow of energy (dashed line) vary directly and are completely in phase.

plate used to demonstrate resistance will be replaced with one that has an insert of airtight but flexible, membranous material, as in Figure 4–5. The membrane is obviously more flexible than the surrounding walls and hence can be stretched into or out of the box as pressure varies. Now study the two waves in Figure 4–6 and imagine the alternate compression and rarefaction of air molecules produced by a sound wave: at a phase of 90 degrees, condensation is at its maximum (point *A*), and at 270 degrees, rarefaction is maximum (point *C*). As point *A* is approached, the air molecules between the speaker and the membrane are compressed until, at 90 degrees, the molecules are maximally compressed, the membrane is maximally distended, and there is no flow of energy. The energy has not been lost, however, as it was in the purely resistive system; it is stored in the membrane and will be returned to the system as the pressure moves from its extremes toward 0. At point *B*, pressure is 0 but is changing toward the rarefaction phase at the maximum rate and there is maximum negative flow of energy. Points *C* and *D* reflect

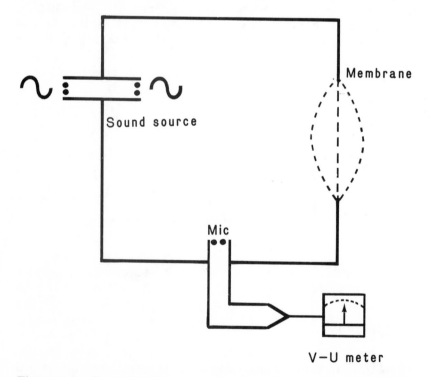

Figure 4–5. One wall of the cavity now has a flexible membrane, responsive to the condensation and rarefaction phases of the constant tone, illustrating the effect of stiffness.

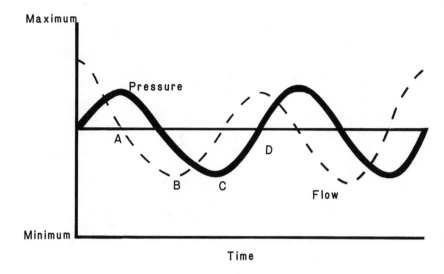

Figure 4-6. When stiffness dominates a vibrating system, pressure and flow are 90° out of phase, with peaks of flow leading peaks of pressure.

the same processes, but with opposite polarity. That is, at C rarefaction is maximum, the membrane is maximally retracted, and again there is no flow of energy. Pressure and flow, therefore, are out of phase with one another; peaks of flow lead peaks of pressure. In a system dominated completely by stiffness, the two factors are 90 degrees out of phase.

Systems characterized by great stiffness store more energy to return to the system and therefore transfer less. Systems with great elasticity store less energy and transfer more. In the ear, the tympanic membrane, the ossicular joints, and the air pressure in the middle ear contribute to stiffness.

Mass (X_m)

Energy flow is affected in yet a third way by mass and an associated property, inertia. In Figure 4-7, one wall of the cavity has been replaced with a plug, the diameter of which fits the box exactly, but this plug is free to slide back and forth without friction. The plug has considerably more mass than the air molecules; therefore, it has greater inertia as well. Inertia means that a body tends to remain at rest until set into motion and to remain in motion until stopped. Energy applied to a system with mass is also stored briefly before being returned, but the mode is different from that associated with stiffness.

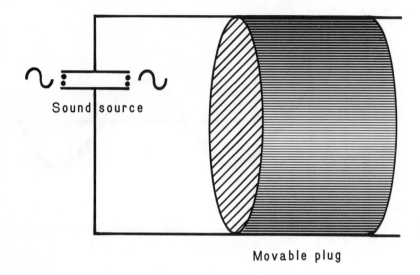

Movable plug

Figure 4–7. A freely movable plug in the cavity demonstrates the effects of mass.

The motion of the plug relative to that of the air particles is delayed as energy is stored in overcoming inertia (Fig. 4–8). By the time the plug finally starts moving in the direction of the pressure wave, the pressure has peaked and is starting to return to 0. The inertia of the mass keeps it in motion until it can be reversed by the opposing force of the pressure wave. If a system is controlled only by mass, there is also a 90 degree phase differential between pressure and flow, but in this case flow lags behind pressure. The mass of the middle ear is determined by its structures (tympanic membrane, ossicles, middle ear mucosa, intratympanic muscles and ligaments) as well as by the density of the fluid or gas occupying its spaces.

The pressure and flow of sound energy, therefore, is affected in predictable ways by three components of the transmitting system—stiffness, mass, and resistance—that together constitute its impedance, expressed in *ohms*. When impedance is high, the flow is low and efficient transmission of sound energy can be maintained only by increasing its pressure, either by increasing the power at the source or by decreasing the volume into which it is directed. When impedance is low, the same amount of energy can be imparted with proportionally lower pressure and higher flow.

The two storage components, mass and stiffness, each characterize *reactance* (X), a term used to predict how a given amount of

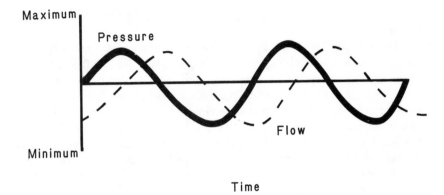

Figure 4–8. In a mass-dominated system, pressure and flow are again 90° out of phase, but peaks of pressure lead peaks of flow.

mass or stiffness will react to sound of different frequency. Stiffness is expressed as *negative* reactance ($-X_c$) and mass as *positive* reactance (X_m) because of the phase relationships of pressure and flow. That is, pressure lags behind flow (is 90 degrees negative) with stiffness and leads flow (is 90 degrees positive) with mass. Therefore, the two terms are 180 degrees out of phase when they influence the same transmitting system. The total reactance (X_t) is simply the algebraic sum of the two quantities. If stiffness predominates, the total reactance will be negative and the converse.

Combined Components

When measurements of middle ear impedance are made at the plane of the tympanic membrane, resistance and reactance components are present simultaneously. Resistance is generated by the transformation of acoustic energy to mechanical energy; and reactance due to both mass and stiffness is characteristic of the tympanic membrane and the enveloped manubrium of the malleus. Resistance and reactance are also affected by the structures and function of the middle ear contents beyond the tympanic membrane. Because of these combined characteristics, when a sound wave encounters the tympanic membrane, part of its energy is lost in the transformation of energy states, part of it is transmitted through the middle ear, and part of it is returned to the system (i.e., reflected back into the ear canal). The ratio of these parts is affected by the frequency of the sound wave interacting with the dominant component (i.e., mass or stiffness reactance) of that ear's acoustic impedance.

The relative contributions of resistance and reactance to middle ear transmission efficiency vary with frequency. At low frequencies, more energy is spent overcoming stiffness; at high frequencies, more energy is spent overcoming the inertial properties of the system's mass. Thus, mass reactance varies directly and stiffness reactance varies inversely with the frequency of the sound being transmitted. Stated another way, the higher the frequency, the greater effect of high mass reactance; and the lower the frequency, the greater effect of high stiffness reactance. Resistance is not affected by frequency.

Since resistance and reactance vary independently of one another with respect to the effect of frequency, they are said to be *orthogonally related*; that is, changes in resistance do not affect the total reactance (or either of its components), and vice versa. Both magnitude and sign (positive or negative) of R and X_t can vary without affecting the other component. Acoustic impedance, however, is the vector sum (not the algebraic sum) of resistance and reactance. A vector is a quantity that can show both magnitude and direction or sign. This means that the total impedance varies under the influence of both resistance and reactance, but that resistance and reactance vary independently. These relationships are illustrated in Figure 4–9. The magnitude of each component is represented by the length of the line. Note first that the total reactance X_t is the algebraic sum of the mass and stiffness reactance shown on the ordinate. In this case (as is usual in human ears) stiffness predominates and therefore the total reactance is negative as well. The resistance, representing the energy dissipated in conversion, is indicated on the abscissa. Because these two terms are at right angles to one another impedance can be calculated according to the Pythagorean principle $c^2 = a^2 + b^2$, or, in this case, $Z^2 = R^2 + X^2$. The equation is simplified to obtain Z:

$$Z = \sqrt{R^2 + X^2}$$

and can then be expanded to show the two parts of reactance:

$$Z = \sqrt{R^2 + (X_m - X_c)^2}$$

The mass reactance at any point in time is calculated as the product of 2π (6.28) times the frequency of the sound times the mass of the system. This is expressed as

$$2\pi f M$$

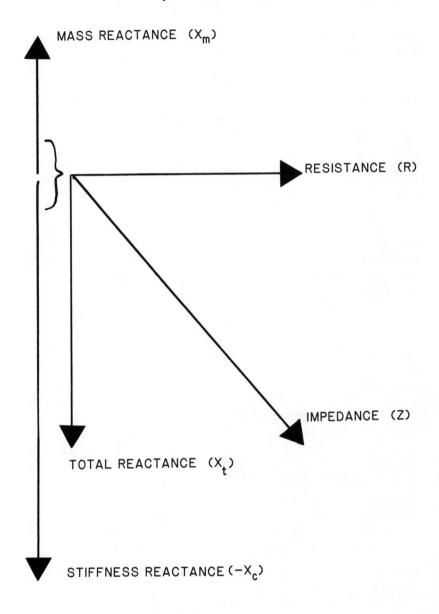

Figure 4–9. The vector sum of resistance and reactance is impedance. Note that resistance and reactance can vary independently but that impedance is affected by both the direction and the magnitude of the two components.

Similarly, the stiffness reactance is calculated as the ratio of the stiffness to 2π times the frequency of the sound, or

$$- k/2\pi f$$

Thus, another way of expressing the following equation would be

$$Z = \sqrt{R^2 + (2\pi f M - k/2\pi f)^2}$$

Berlin and Cullen (1980) provide a fine discussion of the impedance equation and illustrate it with the following example. If the mass of a system is 1 and the frequency of stimulation is 100 Hz, mass reactance is calculated as 628 "mass reactance units" ($X_m = 2\pi f M$ or $2 \times 3.14 \times 100 \times 1 = 628$). The mass reactance term can be increased in two ways: first, by increasing the actual mass; and second, by increasing the frequency. This is illustrated as follows.

Given: Mass of 1	Given: Mass of 2
Frequency: 200 Hz	Frequency: 100 Hz
$X_m = 6.28 \times 200 \times 1$	$X_m = 6.28 \times 100 \times 2$
$X_m = 1256$	$X_m = 1256$

The opposition to a high frequency sound, therefore, varies directly with the mass reactance of the system through which it is transmitted.

The same arbitrary numbers can be used to illustrate the inverse relationship that exists between stiffness reactance and frequency. So, for a stiffness of 1 and a frequency of 100 Hz, the reactance due to stiffness is $1/6.28 \times 100 = 0.000159$ unit of stiffness reactance. Changing the values of stiffness and frequency will again change the value of the reactance:

Given: Stiffness of 1	Given: Stiffness of 2
Frequency: 200 Hz	Frequency: 100 Hz
$X_c = 1/6.28 \times 200$	$X_c = 2/6.28 \times 100$
$X_c = 0.000796$ (1/1256)	$X_c = 0.003318$ (2/628)

Thus, the higher the stiffness of a system, the greater is its opposition to low frequency signals.

A fourth component can be calculated from the expression above: phase angle (Θ). This quantity represents the difference in degrees between the resistance and the total impedance. Figure 4–10 demonstrates that phase angle varies directly with the reactance component and inversely with resistance. Remember that pressure and flow are in phase when only resistance is present, but that pressure and flow are 90 degrees out of phase with reactance.

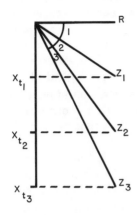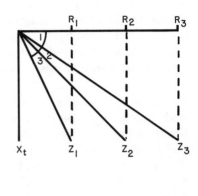

Figure 4-10. Phase angle (Θ) varies directly with the reactance component and inversely with the resistance component of impedance.

Therefore, phase angle is a more convenient way of specifying the difference in time between pressure and flow. For example, the period of a 250 Hz tone is 4 ms; a 90 degree phase differential, therefore, is 1 ms. As the total reactance becomes lower (i.e., as mass and stiffness reactance become more equal), phase angle becomes smaller and there is less difference in time (phase) between pressure and the flow of energy. When total reactance is 0, the transmitting system is at resonance and its total impedance can be accounted for by resistance. In humans, the primary middle ear resonance is at about 1200 Hz, with a smaller resonance near 800 Hz. At frequencies below resonance, the transmitting system is dominated by stiffness reactance; above resonance, the total impedance depends on the mass reactance.

COMPLIANCE AND EQUIVALENT VOLUME

The discussion so far has been concerned with how sound is opposed in its journey through a "system"—the middle ear. The more pertinent question to those who measure auditory function is "How efficient is the ear in transmitting sound when [implicitly] a certain amount of acoustic impedance exists?" This question is concerned with *admittance* (*Y*), or the ease with which the flow of energy can be accomplished in that system. In that sense, admittance is the reciprocal of impedance. Higher impedance results in lower admittance, and lower impedance permits greater admittance. The reciprocal relationship between these two factors has led to widespread use of a new term: *immittance,* representing a morphological blend of impedance and admittance. Immittance, however, should be used with caution because it conveys no direct information about either the impedance or the admittance of the ear and cannot be quantified for use as a clinical or research tool.

In the previous section, it was demonstrated that the amount of opposition to energy flow offered by resistance and both components of reactance can be calculated. The ease with which energy will flow through a system characterized by given amounts of resistance and reactance can also be calculated. *Conductance* is a measure of energy flow through resistance; *susceptance* is a measure of energy flow through reactance. Table 4-1 summarizes these relationships.

Remember that in the middle ear the most influential component of the total impedance—and the most variable—is reactance, most of which can be accounted for by stiffness. Measurement of compliance, therefore, provides a clinically useful indicant of middle ear transmission efficiency.

The compliance of a system is easily expressed in units of cubic centimeters (cc) equivalent volume. "Equivalent" volume? To illustrate this concept, we return to the cavity supplied with a constant sound source and a microphone leading to a sound level meter. Recall that, given a sound source of a constant intensity, sound pressure level varies inversely with cavity volume, as demonstrated in Figure 4-11. This also means that sound pressure level could be predicted by knowing the source intensity and the cavity volume. Larger volumes would predict a lower SPL, and a smaller volume would predict a higher SPL. Again, by keeping sound intensity constant, the cavity volume could be predicted by measuring its sound pressure. A high SPL would predict a small volume, a low SPL a larger volume. All of these examples, however, require the cavity to be acoustically rigid and leakproof.

Now, if the cavity is not leakproof—that is, if some sound could escape—we would find that the sound pressure in the cavity was lower than it should be, given the volume. The sound pressure would be equivalent to that expected in a larger cavity. If we wished to maintain a constant sound pressure in cavities of different volumes, we could do so only by changing the power at the sound source. A smaller cavity would require proportionally less power

Table 4–1.   Relationship Between Impedance and Admittance

Impedance (Z)		Factor	Admittance (Y)	
Units	Terms		Terms	Units
Ohm	Resistance	FRICTION	Conductance	Mho
Ohm	Mass Reactance	MASS	Susceptance	Mho
Ohm	Stiff Reactance	STIFFNESS	Compliance	cc

than a larger one to maintain the sound pressure level criterion.

This analogy can be carried one step further: Figure 4–12 represents a cavity connected by a flexible membrane to a system possessing a certain amount of friction, stiffness, and mass. When sound is introduced into this cavity, the sound pressure will be lower than might be predicted on the basis of its size. This is because some of the energy is lost in overcoming friction, and some of it is transmitted on through the system. The measured sound pressure in the cavity will be largely dependent on how much energy is returned to the system (i.e., reflected back from the membrane). This in turn depends on the stiffness and mass of the system as well as on the frequency of the (source) tone. If very little is reflected, the sound pressure will be lower, meaning that energy has flowed very easily through the system. Conversely, a higher SPL (and a smaller equivalent volume) means energy flow has not been efficient. This would appear to indicate that higher equivalent volume could be equated in a simple way with greater energy flow. Such a conclusion would be inaccurate for two reasons.

First, the equivalent volume is not independent of the actual volume of the cavity; thus, the smaller the actual volume, the higher the SPL produced by a signal of a constant intensity at its source. Less obvious, but equally important, is the fact that an enclosed volume of air has its own impedance—because it has mass in the form of molecules and friction in the form of their random collision—and thus adds to the impedance of another system. The air also has stiffness, which is determined by the size of the cavity. This is something we have all experienced when using a pump to inflate a bicycle tire or other inflatable objects. Operation of the pump is easy in the beginning, but it becomes more and more difficult as the tire fills with air. This indicates that the flow of energy is more difficult through a small volume of air than through a larger one. Finally, the stiffness or elasticity of the enclosed air is affected by such variables as altitude, heat, and humidity, all fac-

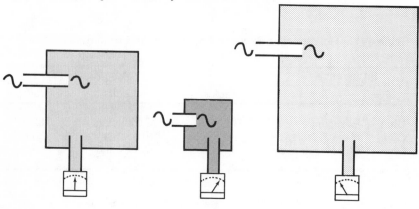

Figure 4–11. The relationship between sound pressure and the volume of an enclosed cavity. As the volume decreases, sound pressure—the force/unit area—increases. As volume is increased, sound pressure decreases.

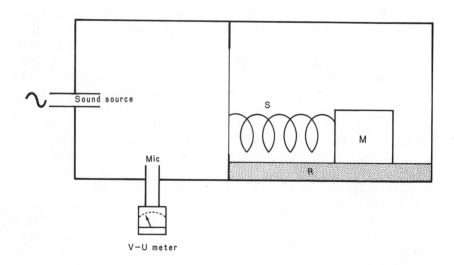

Figure 4–12. Schematic diagram of a vibrating system characterized by the mass (M) of a block, the stiffness (S) of a spring used to move the block, and the resistance (R) of a surface over which the block must move.

tors that influence the mass and density of the air. These factors are important in the interpretation of clinical measurements of compliance.

The development of the electromechanical impedance bridge and later the electroacoustic impedance and the oto-admittance meter, based on the principles presented here, opened a new age in the assessment of auditory function.

ELECTROACOUSTIC IMPEDANCE BRIDGES

Devices used to measure acoustic impedance or admittance are no more intricate in principle than the various models discussed in the previous sections of this chapter. A volume of air is enclosed in the ear canal, thus forming an airtight cavity when the meatus is blocked with a plug. Within the plug are a transducer from a constant sound source and a microphone connected to a sound level meter. One wall of the cavity—the tympanic membrane—is more flexible than the others; it is attached to the middle ear structures that have certain amounts of stiffness, mass, and friction. The measuring device determines the combined effect of these variables on the sound pressure level of the source tone in the cavity.

The earliest impedance meters, such as one designed by Zwislocki (1963), measured acoustic impedance, resistance, and reactance directly. However, the values derived by these devices represented the combined impedance of the middle ear and the air column in the canal when only that of the middle ear was of clinical interest. This problem was resolved by determining actual ear canal volume in each subject: the ear canal was filled with alcohol, which was then drained and its volume measured. In this way, a correction could be made to the impedance measure, resulting in a value that was representative of only the middle ear, and from which the reactance and resistance components could be calculated directly.

Although accurate and reliable in practiced hands, the Zwislocki bridge presented several problems for clinical applications, not the least of which was the inconvenience and mess of measuring ear canal volume with alcohol. Yet, canal volume must be considered if impedance measurements are to be accurate. An ingenious alternative to direct measurement was offered by including an air pressure pump in the design of later electroacoustic impedance bridges.

The earliest part of this chapter showed that the volume of a hard-walled cavity could be determined by measuring the sound pressure level within the cavity of a tone having a known intensity at its source. If the cavity were not completely rigid, however, the sound pressure would be less than predicted by its actual volume, indicating that some of the sound was transmitted out of the cavity. Under ordinary circumstances, the tympanic membrane permits the effective transmission of sound from the ear canal through the middle ear system. By "ordinary circumstances" two conditions are implied: (1) middle ear structures that are intact and functioning normally; and (2) air pressure in the ear canal equal to that within the middle ear cavity. When equal pressures are not maintained across the tympanic membrane, its stiffness is altered. A difference of only 50 mm H_2O between middle ear and ear canal pressure reduces the compliance of the tympanic membrane by 40 to 50 percent (Brooks, 1976). Greater pressure differentials result in further increases in stiffness until, at about ± 200 mm, the tympanic membrane is so loaded that it functions as an acoustically rigid structure, reflecting most sound energy back into the canal. At this point, the equivalent volume is a reasonably good estimate of the actual volume contained within the canal, the impedance of which can then be subtracted from the total to arrive at that of the middle ear.

Figure 4-13 is a schematic diagram of instruments that are designed to measure acoustic compliance. The main feature is the probe tip that contains all the systems necessary to permit such measurements: First, there is a tube that transmits a low frequency tone (the *probe tone*) through a variable gain amplifier to a speaker. Second, there is a tube that is attached to the pressure pump, through which air pressure in the ear canal can be varied. A third tube contains a microphone to receive the sound in the canal.

The sound thus collected is filtered, amplified, rectified (converted from AC to DC voltage), and then conducted to a device called a center balance voltmeter that functions like the old-fashioned scales designed to weigh some material against a standard weight. The ear canal sound voltage is applied to one side of the voltmeter; the other side is supplied with a constant voltage, equal to that which would produce exactly 95 dB SPL in a cavity of a set volume. The sound pressure level of the probe tone in the ear canal is variable and is determined by three factors: (1) the volume of air enclosed between the probe tip and the tympanic membrane; (2) the amount of sound energy supplied to the ear canal through the speaker, which is controlled by the amplifier; and (3) the relative

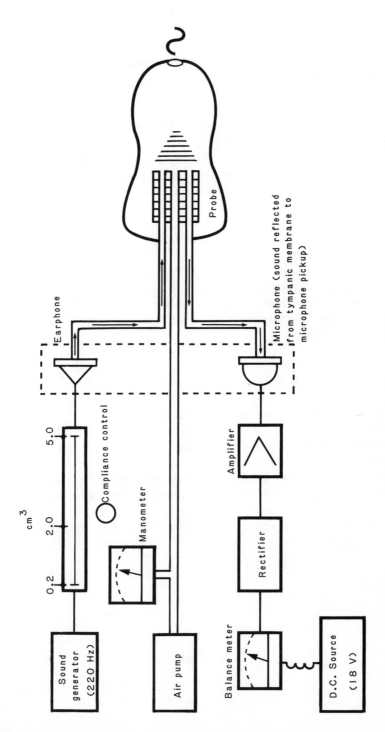

Figure 4–13. Schematic diagram of an electroacoustic impedance meter.

amounts of sound energy absorbed and reflected by the tympanic membrane. Higher sound pressure levels in the canal, therefore, can be achieved either by increasing the energy at its source or by reducing the transmission efficiency at the tympanic membrane. The principle is to keep the voltmeter balanced at 0, with a goal of determining how much sound energy must be directed into the ear canal to maintain voltage equal to that resulting in a sound pressure of 95 dB. If a great amount of sound is reflected from the tympanic membrane, less energy will be required to keep the voltmeter balanced; if more sound is absorbed, proportionally more energy is required. This clever design permits dynamic measurement of middle ear function because a change in compliance at the tympanic membrane for any reason will produce a change in the amount of sound energy needed at the source to maintain the criterion balance on the voltmeter.

The clinical assessment of middle ear function is accomplished by recording acoustic compliance as it is affected by changes in air pressure (tympanometry) and by reflex activity of the intratympanic muscles. The following chapter will consider these applications in some detail.

STUDY QUESTIONS

1. How does impedance relate to admittance?
2. What are the sources of reactance in the ear? Of resistance?
3. What factors determine the SPL of a low frequency probe tone in the ear canal?
4. How does acoustic impedance relate to middle ear resonance?
5. What is immittance? What does it tell us about the status of the middle ear?
6. Why is ear canal volume an important variable in clinical measurement of acoustic impedance or admittance?

Chapter 5

Clinical Applications of Acoustic Immittance

One of the first goals of hearing assessment is to distinguish between conductive and sensorineural impairment. For many years otologists have relied on otoscopic examination and tuning fork tests as a means of obtaining information about middle ear status. Pure tone audiometry, based on the principles of tuning fork tests, offers another way of obtaining such information and can also indicate the severity of an impairment. However, there are some serious limitations to both methods. First, many patients are unable (or unwilling) to cooperate with the test procedures. Second, exact information that can be deduced about the underlying cause of a conductive or sensorineural disorder is limited. Third, there are many sources of error in the measurement of bone conduction that may lead to inaccuracy in categorizing the type and severity of hearing impairment.

These problems have been reduced, although not entirely eliminated, by the use of immittance audiometry. Voluntary responses are not required and therefore subjects can be tested independently of their age, mental status, state of consciousness, or ability to respond. Immittance results can help provide information about the likelihood of a specific condition, differentiate among several possible conditions, and monitor treatment effectiveness. Furthermore, such information is not limited to the mechanical function of the middle ear but can also be used to assess cochlear, auditory nerve, brain stem, and facial nerve integrity. For these reasons, immittance audiometry is the cornerstone of a battery of tests for comprehensive auditory assessment.

The clinical measurement of acoustic immittance is based on three components: (1) determination of static compliance; (2) tympanometry; and (3) measurement of acoustic reflexes.

STATIC COMPLIANCE

We have already discussed, in another context, the concept of static compliance. Recall that the compliance of the middle ear is derived by subtracting the compliance at +200 mm (which represents that of the air column between the probe tip and the tympanic membrane) from the total compliance when pressure is equal on each side of the tympanic membrane and energy transfer is at a peak. Thus,

$$\text{Middle ear compliance} = \text{Peak compliance} - \text{Compliance}_{200\text{mm}}$$
$$MEC = C_{peak} - C_{200}$$

Static compliance is simply another way of describing middle ear compliance. Low static compliance, therefore, indicates that energy transfer is only slightly improved by equalizing pressures across the tympanic membrane. "Normal" static compliance values usually fall in the range of 0.3 to 1.6 cc.

There are several reasons, however, why static compliance measurements are of limited clinical value. First, there is substantial variability among normal individuals when middle ear compliance is measured with the above-mentioned method and therefore the line between "normal" and "abnormal" becomes extremely fuzzy. Second, measured static compliance is most indicative of the status of the tympanic membrane, not of the entire middle ear complex. For this reason, compliance values within the normal range are often obtained from subjects with early stapes fixation or a retracted but normally mobile tympanic membrane. Similarly, abnormally high or low values may indicate nothing more serious than a slightly flaccid or thickened membrane, respectively. Third, the static compliance is influenced not only by the condition of the tympanic membrane and ossicles but also by the volume of air enclosed between the probe tip and the tympanic membrane. As you will recall, a smaller volume of air has greater stiffness than a larger one; therefore, the apparent difference between middle ear compliance and the compliance of the air enclosed in a very small canal may be artificially small, influenced as much by the canal volume as by the actual mechanics of the middle ear. Atmospheric conditions such as altitude, heat, and humidity also influence the stiffness of the air in the canal. For these reasons, static compliance is considered to be the weakest part of the immittance battery and should never form the basis on which clinical decisions are made.

TYMPANOMETRY

A tympanogram is a graphic representation of middle ear compliance under changing pressure conditions. Compliance (in cc equivalent volume) is shown on the ordinate, and relative pressure (in mm H_2O) is plotted on the abscissa. What is meant by "relative pressure"? Recall that acoustic transmission is most efficient when air pressure in the middle ear cavity is the same as ambient (atmospheric) pressure. Atmospheric pressure, of course, varies with geographic locale—Denver, at a high altitude, has lower atmospheric pressure than San Diego, which is at sea level—and to some extent with weather conditions. Thus, "0 mm" means only that the air pressure produced in the ear canal is the same as ambient pressure—there is 0 difference. A reading of +50 mm means that canal air pressure is 50 mm greater than ambient, whereas −50 mm means that canal pressure is 50 mm less than ambient. Air pressure can also be measured in pascals (Pa), by 1 mm of water where pressure (1 mm H_2O) is equivalent to about 10 Pa or 1 deca Pascal (daPa). Therefore, 100 mm H_2O = 100 daPa, 200 mm H_2O = 200 daPa, and so forth.

Remember than when equal pressures are not maintained across the tympanic membrane, its stiffness is altered. As pressure increases, more and more of the probe tone is reflected from the drum surface, causing an increase in sound pressure level in the canal and a corresponding decrease of the equivalent volume. A normal pressure-compliance function, therefore, would show proportionally lower equivalent volume at high positive and negative pressures, increasing as pressure approaches the 0, or the equalization point. Such a function is shown in Figure 5-1.

The shape of the pressure-compliance function is altered in some rather predictable ways by various middle ear abnormalities,

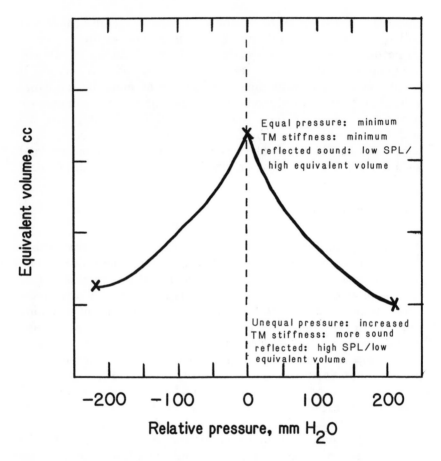

Equal pressure: minimum TM stiffness: minimum reflected sound: low SPL/ high equivalent volume

Unequal pressure: increased TM stiffness: more sound reflected: high SPL/low equivalent volume

Relative pressure, mm H$_2$O

Figure 5-1. A normal pressure-compliance function. As ear canal pressure approximates middle ear pressure, more sound is accepted by the middle ear, leading to a larger equivalent volume.

although, as we shall see, the effects are by no means invariant. Tympanograms are classified with respect to the following factors: (1) shape of the function (peaked, flat, rounded, etc.); (2) location of the compliance peak; and (3) the difference in compliance between the value at +200 mm H$_2$O and that at the peak (static compliance). Three major categories and two subcategories of tympanograms have been described by Jerger (1970) and are in common clinical usage by many who conduct immittance measurements using a low frequency probe tone, such as 220 Hz. When a higher frequency probe tone is used, variations in these patterns can be expected.

Type A

The Type A pattern is characterized by a *clear peak* that occurs at *0 mm ±50 mm*, as shown in Figure 5–2. All three Type A tympanograms share these two characteristics. The base-peak compliance difference is in the range of 0.3 to 1.6 cc.

This pattern is usually seen in subjects with normal middle ear function, although it is not uncommonly found with early stapes fixation. It is important to understand that a tympanogram is a test only of eardrum and ossicle mobility, not a test of hearing sensitivity. Even persons with the most profound deafness show Type A tympanograms if middle ear function is normal.

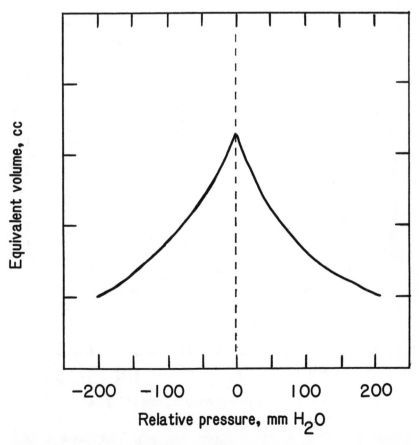

Figure 5–2. Type A tympanogram. Note peak compliance at 0 mm and base-peak compliance in the range of 0.3 to 1.6 cc.

Type A$_S$

Like the Type A, the Type A$_S$ pattern has a definable peak compliance at normal atmospheric pressure (i.e., 0 mm or 0 Pa). However, the base-peak compliance difference is low—under 0.3 cc (Fig. 5–3). The subscript "s," therefore, refers to the shallow curve representing an abnormally stiff mechanism. Recall that the effect of increasing stiffness is to make transmission of low frequency signals (such as the probe tone) less efficient. If stiffness is increased, the probe tone will be poorly transmitted, with more reflected back from the tympanic membrane. Therefore, compliance is low and is changed only slightly by equalization of pressure across the tympanic membrane. This pattern may result from a variety of pathological conditions, such as thickened tympanic membrane, adhesions, and ossicular fixation.

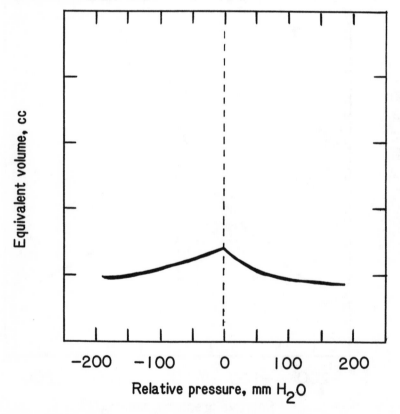

Figure 5-3. Type A$_S$ tympanogram. The peak compliance at 0mm ± 50mm demonstrates normal middle ear pressure; the low base-peak compliance suggests increased stiffness loading of the middle ear structures.

Type A_d

In contrast to the usually shallow A_s pattern, the Type A_d is characterized by unusually high compliance in the 0 mm area. Therefore, it is often described as a deep tympanogram, which can signal ossicular discontinuity. Compliance is so great that it may exceed the limits of the equipment, as in Figure 5–4. This is a situation in which high compliance is not synonymous with highly effective transmission. The A_d pattern commonly appears when the patient has a very flaccid tympanic membrane, produced by widespread atrophic scarring on its surface. The distinction between such a relatively benign condition and the more serious ossicular disruption is helped by knowing (1) the patient's history; (2) the otoscopic appearance of the tympanic membrane; (3) the status of the acoustic reflexes in the affected ear; and (4) pure tone audiometric results.

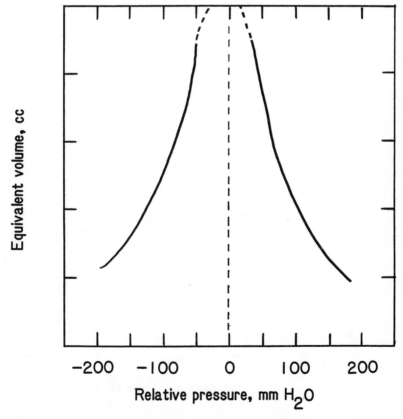

Figure 5–4. Type A_d tympanogram. Normal middle ear pressure is present, but there is abnormally high compliance (flaccidity) in the system.

Type B

The most unequivocally abnormal tympanometric pattern is the Type B (Fig. 5–5). In this type there is little or no effect of pressure change on the compliance of the tympanic membrane; thus, the pressure-compliance function shows no peak but defines more of a straight line. This means that the probe tone has encountered a relatively immovable barrier and is being poorly transmitted through the middle ear. Although the Type B is most closely associated with the presence of serous otitis media, a number of other conditions will yield this pattern as well. The key to distinguishing among these conditions lies in considering both the shape of the tympanogram and the equivalent volume.

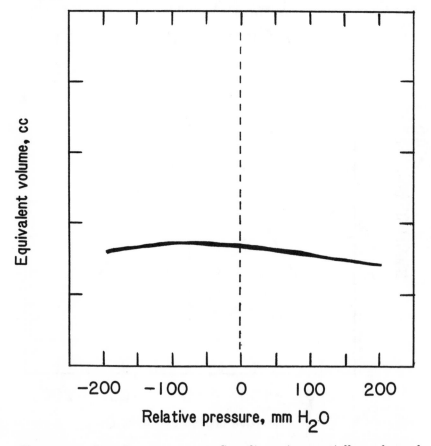

Figure 5–5. Type B tympanogram. Compliance is essentially unchanged by ear canal pressure variations; there is no identifiable peak.

Impacted Cerumen. When a mass of cerumen is situated in the ear canal in such a way as to block the tympanic membrane, two results are seen. First, the size of the hard-walled cavity is reduced to the space between the probe tip and the cerumen. This results in an inappropriately small equivalent volume (see Fig. 5–6). Second, the cerumen mass has much higher impedance than that of the tympanic membrane or middle ear structures—so great that it is affected inconsequentially by the air pressures applied in clinical tympanometry. The Type B pattern in this case, therefore, is characterized by very low equivalent volume with little or no change in compliance across the pressure range. It is hoped, of course, that preliminary otoscopic inspection of the ear canal and drum will have alerted the examiner to that possibility. There should be no

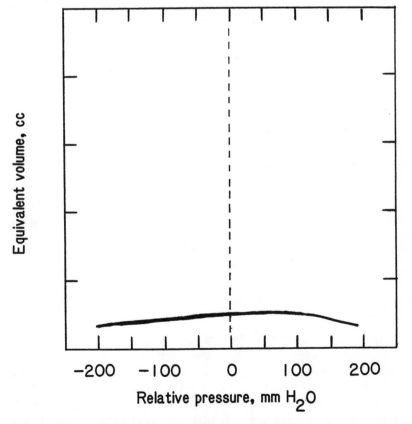

Figure 5-6. A Type B tympanogram is produced by a plug of impacted cerumen (a) by reducing the volume of the cavity to that contained between the probe tip and the plug and (b) by the greater mass of the plug, which is not affected by the pressure variations in the ear canal.

attempt on the part of nonphysicians to remove material from a patient's ear canal; medical referral is necessary.

Foreign Bodies. The variety of objects that can be introduced into the ear canal is limited only by people's imaginations and by the size of the object. If the canal were completely occluded by a foreign body, the tympanogram would resemble that seen with impacted cerumen, for the same reasons. However, tympanometry should *not* be attempted in this circumstance; prompt medical referral for removal of the foreign body is indicated.

Canal Wall Placement of Probe Tip. The external ear canal follows an S-shaped course that is more tortuous in some individuals than in others. Unless the probe tip is inserted into the canal along that course, it will come to rest against one of the canal walls. In this case, the volume between the probe tip and the canal wall is quite small and the majority of the probe tone is reflected. Therefore, the tympanogram shows an exceedingly small equivalent volume, with little or no change in compliance. This is a very common problem encountered by inexperienced examiners, second only to failure to achieve an airtight seal.

If otoscopic examination has shown the ear canal to be free of obstruction and a tympanic membrane with normal landmarks, a Type B tympanogram with small equivalent volume—especially in adults—means the examiner should remove and replace the probe, then repeat the tympanogram.

Middle Ear Effusion. In this situation the middle ear space is occupied by some liquid or semiliquid material. Any liquid has a higher impedance than air; hence, more probe tone is reflected, resulting in low compliance. When positive pressure is applied, the liquid cannot be compressed and there is little or no change in compliance. Similarly, when negative pressure is applied, the fluid expands to fill the available space, and again compliance is unchanged.

Tympanic Membrane Perforation. Some clinicians feel that tympanometry should not be attempted when a perforation is known to exist because of the slight danger of infection. Occasionally, however, a perforation is not visible because of its size or location. In this instance, a Type B tympanogram will appear, showing a large equivalent volume and little or no change in compliance across the pressure range. How is this pattern produced? Recall that the equivalent volume of the cavity with an applied pressure of +200 mm H_2O is an effective estimate of the volume between the probe tip and the tympanic membrane. The greater the distance between these two points, the greater the equivalent volume. If the tympanic membrane is perforated, the volume of the middle ear cleft and mastoid air cell system (an average of 2 cc) is added to the volume of the ear canal. Thus, a large equivalent volume is shown. This is demonstrated in Figure 5–7. When air pressure is applied through the probe tip, it is vented into the middle ear space through the perforation and thus the compliance of the tympanic membrane is unchanged. If the eustachian tube is functional, positive pressure

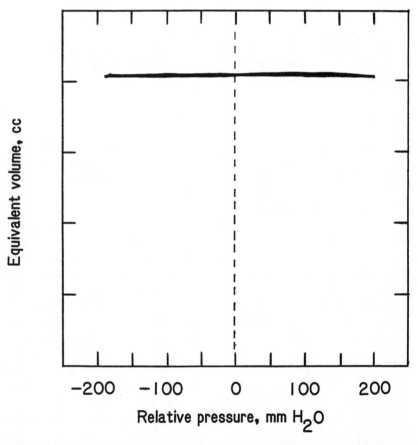

Figure 5–7. A Type B tympanogram typically produced by a tympanic membrane perforation or by a patent pressure-equalizing tube. Note the large equivalent volume, representing the combined volume of the ear canal and middle ear space.

can be maintained only briefly before it is equalized, whereas both positive and negative pressure is held when the eustachian tube is blocked.

Intact Tympanostomy (Pressure-Equalizing) Tubes. The use of "PE" tubes in the management of chronic serous or secretory otitis media is quite common. An incision is made in the tympanic membrane, the fluid is removed, and small grommet tubes are inserted to (1) keep the "perforation" open and (2) allow aeration of the middle ear. When the tubes are patent (i.e., when they allow air to move freely in and out of the middle ear space), tympanometry results are essentially identical to those obtained when a naturally occurring perforation is present. If the tubes are occluded, however, a Type B tympanogram with low to average equivalent volume may be seen, representing only that space between the probe tip and the tympanic membrane. This differentiation is helpful in monitoring the integrity of the tubes when clear visualization of the tympanic membrane is not possible.

Type C

The Type C tympanogram is a clear sign that some kind of eustachian tube malfunction is present because middle ear pressure is at least 100 mm lower than ambient pressure. This pattern, shown in Figure 5–8, is characterized by a peak compliance that is found in the negative range relative to normal; that is, when middle ear pressure is low relative to ambient pressure, peak compliance can be achieved only by setting the pressure in the canal equal to that in the middle ear. At other pressure conditions, the tympanic membrane is stiffened and thus acts as an inefficient transmitter of the low frequency probe tone. If pressure imbalance is the only middle ear problem, the base-peak compliance usually falls in the normal range of 0.3 to 1.6 cc. A Type C pattern usually precedes the development of a Type B pattern owing to serous otitis media, just as it demonstrates recovery as air replaces fluid in the middle ear. For this reason, tympanometry can be useful in monitoring the status of otitis-prone individuals and in assessing treatment effectiveness. Serial tympanograms illustrating this application are shown in Figure 5–9. What does the Type C pattern tell us about middle ear function?

Air is constantly absorbed by the tissue lining the middle ear space. When air is not regularly replaced in the middle ear through the eustachian tube (or a PE tube) but the process of absorption

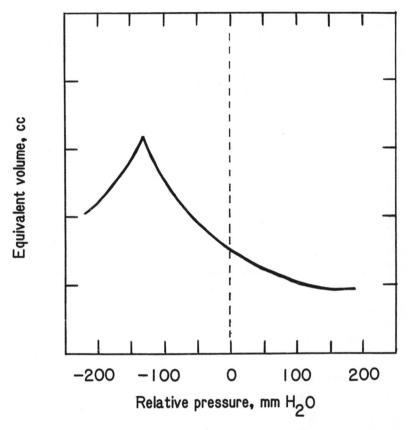

Figure 5-8. Type C tympanogram. Note that base-peak compliance is within normal limits (0.3 to 1.6 cc) but that the peak of the function is shifted into the negative range.

continues, air pressure in the middle ear is reduced and a vacuum begins to develop. As this happens, the tympanic membrane becomes more and more retracted and its stiffness is thereby increased. This means that the low frequency probe tone is poorly transferred into the middle ear; more is reflected back into the canal, resulting in a low equivalent volume. Refer to the series of tympanograms in Figure 5-9. Notice that the ear canal volume remains essentially constant (+ 200 mm) while equivalent volume at 0 mm becomes smaller as the peak moves farther into the negative range. Continued lack of aeration results in the secretion of fluid: peak compliance lessens and the peak eventually disappears as fluid fills the middle ear, producing the Type B. For a more com-

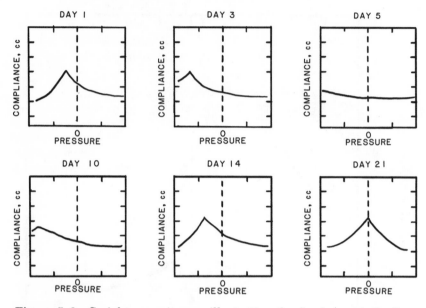

Figure 5-9. Serial tympanograms illustrating the development of a Type B tympanogram during an episode of serous otitis media and a return to normal middle ear status after treatment.

plete discussion of this process, the reader is referred to Bluestone's chapter on the topic (1980).

Other Patterns

The foregoing classification scheme and its association with middle ear disorders depends largely on the use of a low frequency probe tone that is sensitive to changes in the elastic reactance of the middle ear. The acoustic consequences of middle ear pathology are not limited to changes in stiffness, however. The resonant frequency of the middle ear, for example, becomes higher with ossicular fixation and lower with ossicular discontinuity. Similarly, a middle ear tumor such as cholesteatoma greatly increases the contribution of mass to the total impedance. Therefore, it should not be too surprising that higher frequency probe tones (660 to 800 Hz) produce tympanograms of different appearance with certain middle ear disorders.

The most commonly reported abnormal tympanogram produced with a higher frequency probe tone is one having a double peak or "W" shape in the area of maximum compliance. This pattern has been associated with ossicular discontinuity, with flaccidity or scarring on the tympanic membrane, and with areas of retraction limited to the pars flaccida of the tympanic membrane (Brooks, 1976).

An assessment of middle ear function should not be limited to tympanometry, even for purposes of screening. If it is, the potential for errors is very great; "normal" tympanograms can occur in the presence of significant middle ear pathology, and "abnormal" tympanograms can occur when middle ear status is essentially normal with respect to its sound-conducting properties. The measurement of acoustic reflexes offers a method of cross-checking the mechanical function of the middle ear and opens a broad window onto possible sources of peripheral and central auditory dysfunction.

ACOUSTIC REFLEXES

Mechanisms and Characteristics

The middle ear contains two small muscles: the tensor tympani, connected to the malleus; and the stapedius, attached to the stapes. These muscles contract reflexively to certain acoustic and tactile stimuli; in doing so they increase the stiffness of the middle ear. Such an increase means that acoustic impedance is increased; that is, more opposition is offered to the flow of energy. Consequently, the transmission characteristics of the middle ear are altered: because stiffness is increased, low frequencies are transmitted less efficiently. This in effect creates a high-pass filter and raises middle ear resonant frequency. Therefore, the muscles can be viewed as the effectors or regulators of an acoustic input control system to the cochlea. Because the stapedius contracts most consistently to acoustic stimuli, its action has come to be known as the acoustic reflex. Most researchers agree that it is the stapedius (rather than the tensor tympani) that is responsible for the dynamic properties of the acoustic reflex, and the discussion will proceed on that assumption.

In an earlier chapter we discussed principles underlying the design and operation of electroacoustic impedance bridges (see Fig. 4-13). Recall that a key feature of an impedance bridge is a balancing voltmeter that compares sound pressure level in the ear canal with a reference value for the same volume. Changes in immittance at the tympanic membrane disturb that balance and enable the measurement of acoustic compliance on the basis of equivalent volume. Acoustic reflexes are evoked by presenting a sufficiently intense activator signal to the subject by means of a standard earphone on the ear opposite to the probe or through the probe itself. When the reflex occurs, the middle ear is stiffened, leading to inefficient transmission of low frequency sounds (the probe tone) and a subsequent increase in canal SPL as more tone is reflected from the tympanic membrane. This creates an imbalance on the voltmeter, which continues until the reflex has ended. It is very important to keep a clear distinction in your mind between the *activator tone,* which is used to evoke the reflex, and the *probe tone,* which is used to measure the effects of the reflex.

Look at the waveform in Figure 5–8. It represents the change in acoustic immittance caused by contraction of the stapedius muscle. That change can be described in three basic ways. First, the *magnitude* or *amplitude* of the change can be measured in ohms (impedance), mho (admittance), cc equivalent volume (compliance), or dB attentuation of the probe tone. Second, the time in milliseconds (ms) from the onset of the stimulus to some criterion point along the

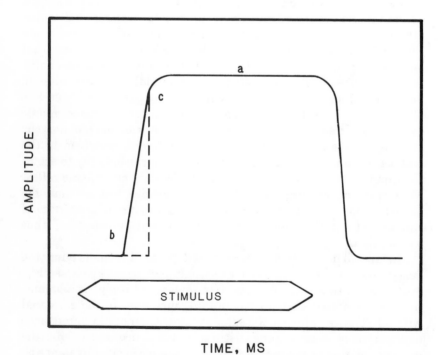

TIME, MS

Figure 5–10. Acoustic reflex waveform and its associated parameters of amplitude (A), onset latency (B), and rise time (C).

response waveform—its *latency*—can be measured. Third, the *rise time* of the response, or the time needed to achieve 90 to 100 percent of the full amplitude from a baseline point can be determined. Reflex amplitude, latency, and rise time are affected in different ways by various stimulus and subject variables, but the clinical utility of these characteristics has only begun to be explored. Most clinical studies have been based on acoustic reflex thresholds and on changes in amplitude over time.

Reflex threshold to a given stimulus can be defined in two broad ways: first, as the intensity necessary to elicit a change in stapedius electromyographic activity (the electric muscle potentials), which signals contraction of muscle fibers; and second, as the intensity required to produce a change in the immittance of the ear. The first measure is a direct indication whereas the second is indirect, occurring as a consequence of stapedius muscle activity, but separated in time and space from the physiological event. Use of the indirect method assumes that the change in immittance produced by stapedius contraction is measurable. Therefore, the middle ear structures must be capable of transmitting such a change to the tympanic membrane, and the measuring equipment must be sensitive enough to record it.

Acoustic reflexes can be elicited in response to a wide range of acoustic stimuli, including clicks, tones, noise, and speech. In all cases, the stimuli must be presented at levels greater than the individual's auditory threshold for that stimulus. In normal subjects, bilaterally symmetrical acoustic reflexes appear at about 85 to 100 dB SPL for tones and at some 10 to 15 dB lower for complex stimuli such as noise bands or speech. In most clinical settings, the level at which the first measurable change in baseline compliance occurs in response to a stimulus is designated "reflex threshold."

The recorded "threshold" can be influenced by a number of nonpathological factors, such as the sensitivity of the measuring instrument and its inherent noise, the step size (5 dB versus 1 dB) and duration of the stimulus used to search for threshold, and the tester's criterion for and method of detecting immittance changes (e.g., visual or pen-recorded). A complete discussion of these and other factors affecting acoustic reflex thresholds has been written by Gelfand (1984) and is recommended for further study.

The clinical application of acoustic reflex measurements is based on an understanding of some basic physiological mechanisms underlying the generation of acoustic reflexes. Therefore, we will consider characteristics of a reflex arc as they apply to the auditory system.

A reflex arc is one of the simplest neural mechanisms known. Reflexes underlie many familiar experiences: lifting a finger from a hot stove; coughing from a throat irritant; blinking the eyes to avoid injury to them. These reflexes have in common three components: (1) a *sensory or afferent part*; (2) an *interneuron*; and (3) a *motor or efferent part.* The reflex arc defines the location within the central and peripheral nervous system of each of these parts.

The first requirement for a reflex is a receptor that is sensitive to an adequate stimulus. If, for any reason, that requirement is not fully met the afferent part of the arc cannot be activated. For example, the stimulus is inadequate when a middle ear disorder causes an impedance mismatch, which in turn attenuates the stimulus delivered to the cochlea. In the case of sensorineural disorders, a different situation exists: the stimulus may be adequate but meet with inadequate numbers of sensitive receptors. The effect is the same in each case—a failure to activate the afferent portion of the reflex mechanism—but the basis for the failure is different. The sensory part of the acoustic reflex arc, therefore, demands integrity of the middle ear, cochlea, and eighth cranial nerve.*

The second requirement of a reflex is an interneuron or series of neurons capable of relaying information between the sensory and motor nuclei in the nervous system. Borg (1973) has published the most detailed description of the acoustic reflex arc (schematized in Figure 5-11) based on his work in rabbit. Some recent evidence (Thompson, 1983) suggests that the reflex pathways in humans may differ slightly from those described in rabbit and cat. However, clinical data indicate that the interneuron lies in an area delimited by the cochlear nuclei and the superior olivary complexes in the brain stem medulla. This knowledge is of particular importance in interpreting patterns of acoustic reflex abnormality.

The primary, or first-order, neuron extends from the spiral ganglion in the cochlea to the cochlear nucleus, where it synapses. The system then divided into pathways that are *represented both ipsilaterally and contralaterally.* This means that stimulation of *one* ear causes stapedius muscle contraction in *both* ears. An "ipsilateral" reflex is one in which motor activity occurs in the stimulated ear; a "contralateral" reflex means that the motor activity occurs in the ear opposite that stimulated. Thus, four reflexes can be described: one ipsilateral and one contralateral for each ear. As you will see in

---

*Jerger and colleagues (in press) recently demonstrated that acoustic reflexes could be elicited in profoundly deaf persons by direct electrical stimulation of the auditory nerve. However, that is a very special case and will not be considered further here.

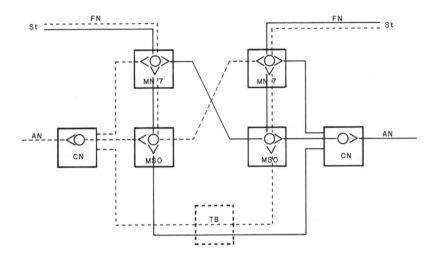

Figure 5-11. Schematic diagram of the acoustic reflex arc. Solid lines indicate right ear pathways, dashed lines indicate left ear pathways. AN: auditory nerve (cranial nerve VIII). CN: cochlear nucleus. TB: trapezoid body. MSO: medial superior olivary complex. MN7: motor nucleus of cranial nerve VII. FN: facial nerve (cranial nerve VII). St: stapedius muscle.

a later section, this feature makes it very convenient to measure acoustic reflexes and provides invaluable clinical information. If you study the schema of the reflex arc, you will see that there are several parallel pathways for each reflex; this arrangement seems to form a fairly robust network that would be difficult to interrupt altogether without relatively extensive damage to the area. When such damage is present, however, sensory information from the periphery cannot be relayed in a normal way to the motor neuron.

The third requirement, completion of the stapedius reflex arc, requires an intact effector mechanism composed of both the muscle and its innervation through the facial nerve (seventh cranial nerve). It is possible for acoustic reflexes to be intact, however, in the presence of significant facial nerve pathology so long as the pathological lesion lies distal (peripheral) to the branch of the facial nerve that innervates the stapedius muscle. The middle ear structures must also be considered a part of the effector mechanism because acoustic reflexes are studied clinically by measuring changes in acoustic immittance, not stapedius muscle contractions.

Acoustic Reflex Abnormalities

How is the acoustic reflex affected by conditions that disrupt the structures or function of the reflex arc? The most conspicuous abnormality is the "absence" of one or more of the four reflexes (right contralateral and ipsilateral, left contralateral and ipsilateral). By "absence" we mean that a measurable change in immittance cannot be monitored when activators are presented at maximum stimulation levels. Taken in isolation, however, this finding is *completely nonspecific*: reflex absence can be a sign of middle ear disorders, severe cochlear disorders, and retrocochlear disorders involving the auditory nerve or brain stem. To account for absent reflexes we must consider (1) the status of all four reflexes, to locate the disorder along the reflex arc; (2) other immittance results, to provide supporting evidence of a middle ear disorder; and (3) the severity and type of pure tone sensitivity loss.

A second (and equally nonspecific) abnormality is represented by elevated reflex threshold. By "elevated" is meant thresholds over 100 dB HL. The significance of an elevated reflex threshold is governed by the type and degree of hearing impairment present. For example, elevated reflex thresholds are common among individuals with mild middle ear disorder because that condition acts to attenuate the activator signal; the amount of threshold elevation then demonstrates the amount of attenuation. Sensorineural hearing loss greater than 60 dB produces the same effect, as do retrocochlear disorders. Again, the results of pure tone audiometry and tympanometry will help to determine the significance of an elevated reflex threshold.

Third, reflex adaptation (or "reflex decay") may occur. This means that the amplitude of an acoustic reflex declines to less than 50 percent of its original amplitude during the presentation of a sustained tone. This phenomenon is illustrated and compared with a normal response in Figure 5–12. Reflex adaptation occurs normally when activator tones over 1000 Hz are used; however, adaptation to a lower frequency tone during the standard 10 s presentation interval is considered an abnormality characteristic of retrocochlear eighth nerve or brain stem disorder. The mechanisms underlying abnormal reflex adaptation are not clear but cannot be accounted for by stapedius muscle fatigue only (Wilson, Shanks, and Lilly, 1984).

Other types of reflex abnormalities have been described in relation to various peripheral and central auditory disorders. These include abnormally low reflex thresholds (<65 dB) for tones; reduced reflex amplitude or amplitude growth; and prolonged onset

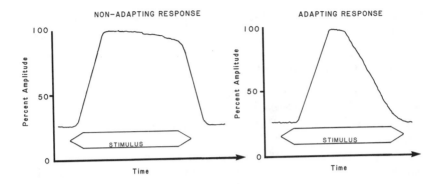

Figure 5-12. Acoustic reflex adaptation, characterized by reduction of reflex amplitude by ≥50 percent within a continuous 10 second period of stimulation.

or offset latency. Although the reliability and clinical usefulness of these measures per se have not been established, they are useful for comparing interaural symmetry and symmetry between ipsilateral and contralateral responses.

Abnormalities of the acoustic reflex are not invariably present with auditory disorders; their appearance, however, provides strong evidence that some part of the reflex mechanism is not functioning normally. In the following section we discuss how a comparison of the status of contralateral and ipsilateral reflexes both permits inferences about the site of auditory disorder and guides the development of a test strategy for the remainder of the assessment.

Patterns of Acoustic Reflex Abnormality

A comparison of the status of the crossed and uncrossed acoustic reflexes, based on an understanding of the reflex arc, allows us to infer a great deal about auditory function at several levels. By applying some simple logic, the status of each reflex can be accounted for.

To observe a normal acoustic reflex, several biological preconditions must be met:

- Stapedius muscles must be intact
- The facial nerve (seventh cranial nerve) must be intact through the level of the branch to the stapedius muscle
- Middle ear function must be normal in each ear
- Sensitivity must be better than about 80 dB HL at the test frequencies

- The auditory nerve (eighth cranial nerve) function must be normal

- Brain stem structures and function must be intact through the level of the olivary nuclei

If one or more of these preconditions are not met, reflex characteristics such as amplitude, threshold, latency, time course, interaural symmetry, and ipsilateral-contralateral symmetry may be altered.

Jerger and Jerger (1977) have used a simple graphic method of comparing crossed and uncrossed reflexes. Their method has been adapted for purposes of this discussion in Figure 5–13. Note first that the location of the probe is used as an anchor point. Thus, R and L mean, respectively, that the probe tip is located in the right ear and in the left ear. The top row represents the status of the crossed, or contralateral, reflex, whereas the bottom represents the status of the uncrossed, or ipsilateral, reflex.

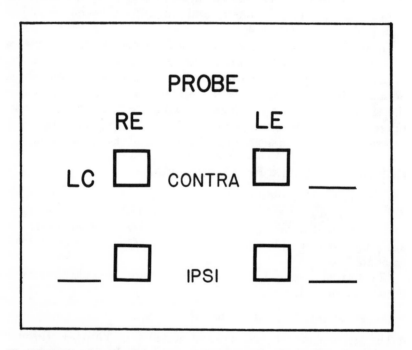

Figure 5–13. Scheme for representing acoustic reflex status. The location of the probe device in the right ear (RE) or left ear (LE) is used as the anchor; the top row depicts the contralateral reflexes (RC, LC); the lower row depicts the ipsilateral reflexes (RI, LI).

It is essential to remember that any reflex must be initiated by a sensory event that activates the afferent part of the reflex arc. Therefore, when the probe tip is located in the right ear, the contralateral reflex shown in the top row means that the left ear has received an activator stimulus. That is, the *test ear* (for purposes of assessing the status of the AR) is the *ear that receives an activator signal.* The top left-hand box, therefore, can be labeled *LC* (left contralateral). This notation tells us that the left ear is stimulated but that the reflex is measured contralaterally in the right ear. Thus, this notation can be used to determine which ear has contributed to the afferent and which has contributed to the efferent portions of a given reflex: The first letter (*R* or *L*) designates the stimulated ear, where the arc begins, and the second letter (*C* or *I*) designates the location of the effector (muscle) relative to the receptor (cochlea). Using this notation, label the other three boxes as *RC, RI,* and *LI.*

For the moment, we will classify acoustic reflexes as normal or abnormal. This simple classification lends itself to illustration of the major reflex patterns among the two ipsilateral and two contralateral reflexes. For this purpose, a shaded box will denote abnormality or absence of the reflex, and an open box will denote normal function.

The Diagonal Pattern

In this pattern (Fig. 5–14) an abnormality is seen to exist on the right contralateral (RC) and right ipsilateral (RI) reflexes. How can we account for this abnormality? To answer this question, recall the preconditions to a normal reflex.

First, there is evidence that the *stapedius muscles are intact bilaterally* because a reflex can be observed both when the probe is in the right ear (LC) and when it is in the left ear (LI). Similarly, *facial nerve function must be adequate* bilaterally to produce contraction of the muscles. The presence of a normal reflex under both probe and earphone configurations also leads to the conclusion that *middle ear function is reasonably normal* in each ear. These series of deductions allow a disorder on the descending (efferent) portion of the reflex arc to be ruled out as an account for the two abnormal reflexes.

The diagonal pattern of reflex abnormality also suggests that a midline disorder at the level of the crossing fibers (a decussation) in the medulla of the brain stem is unlikely. A midline disturbance would affect both crossed reflexes rather than just one; furthermore, an isolated lesion above the decussation would not affect the ipsila-

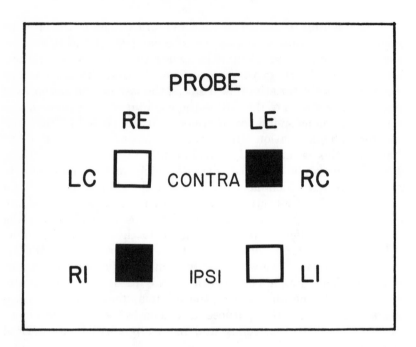

Figure 5-14. The diagonal reflex pattern. Reflexes are abnormal with sound to the affected ear, independent of the location of the probe. This is a "sound effect."

teral reflex in this way. Thus, *brain stem function at the crossing level seems intact.*

Recall that the four reflexes were labeled in such a way as to show which afferent and which efferent system has produced any given reflex. In the present example, the abnormalities are on RC and RI. That is, when the activator is directed to the right ear, a reflex abnormality appears independently of which ear is being used to observe the reflex. This finding implicates the ascending (afferent) system, either peripherally in the cochlea, or centrally in the eighth nerve or cochlear nucleus. For these reasons, the pattern is said to represent a *sound effect.*

The possibility always exists that an abnormal test result is related to faulty test equipment. Routine and frequent listening checks of the equipment, in addition to regular output calibration, can minimize the likelihood that a mechanical failure (such as a "dead" earphone) will go undetected. In the present example, since the earphone signal elicits a normal reflex when on the left ear (LC) and the probe does so as well when it is in the left ear (LI), an external factor seems unlikely.

The diagonal pattern appears when there is severe to profound sensitivity loss on the test ear or when there is a retrocochlear eighth nerve disorder. The reflex pattern, therefore, cannot and should not be used by itself as an indicant of any one type of disorder without confirmation by another independent, converging measure. Obviously, if pure tone testing shows sensitivity better than 80 dB HL, the possibility of a retrocochlear disorder must be seriously considered.

The Horizontal Pattern

In this situation, an abnormality appears on each crossed reflex while the two ipsilateral reflexes remain intact bilaterally (Fig. 5–15). Using the same logic as in the diagonal pattern, we can conclude the following:

- Stapedius muscles are intact bilaterally (reflexes appear with probe right and probe left)

- Facial nerve function is intact bilaterally through the stapedius branch (reflexes appear with probe right and probe left)

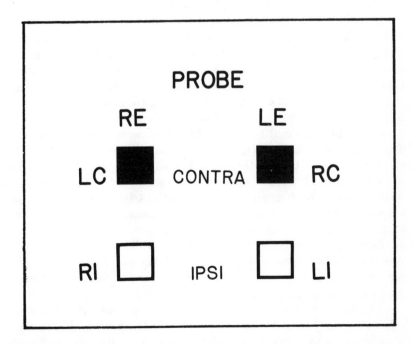

Figure 5–15. The horizontal reflex pattern. Only contralateral reflexes are abnormal.

- Middle ear function is intact bilaterally (reflexes appear with probe and sound right and with probe and sound left)
- There is adequate sensitivity and adequate eighth nerve function bilaterally (reflexes appear with sound right and sound left)

Although the horizontal pattern is generally regarded as the unique signature of a brain stem disorder involving the trapezoid body or the superior olivary complexes, or both, the clinician must be alert to the possibility of a horizontal pattern developing as a result of collapsing ear canals or a weak earphone. Once these external factors can be ruled out, appropriate tests should be carried out to further investigate the likelihood of retrocochlear brain stem disorder.

The Vertical Pattern

Recall that the diagonal pattern was produced by a *sound effect*—that is, an abnormality appeared when the activator sound was directed to a particular ear. The vertical pattern is produced by a *probe effect*—that is, the abnormality appears only when the probe is in a particular ear, as in Figure 5–16.

In this case, we cannot account for the abnormal reflexes on the basis of an afferent disorder; a reflex is present when sound is directed to both the left ear (LC) and the right ear (RI). There is no sound effect. The presence of a normal crossed reflex (LC) shows that the midline crossing fibers in the brain stem are intact. Having ruled out a sound effect and a crossing effect leaves three possibilities to account for a probe effect in this pattern.

First, an abnormality of the stapedius muscle may be present. The patient may have no stapedius muscle on the probe side. This can occur congenitally, although it is quite rare: the odds of having a congenitally absent stapedius muscle are about 1 in 3,000,000. A more common reason why the reflex might be absent is that the stapedius tendon was surgically divided, usually in the course of a stapedectomy. This can be determined by the history.

Second, a peripheral facial nerve disorder may exist. If so, a unilateral facial weakness or total paralysis will be evident. Such a disorder, previously unidentified, must always result in prompt medical referral.

Third, a mild middle ear disorder may be present. As Jerger and colleagues (1974) and later Lutman (1984) showed, the probe is uniquely sensitive to even slight changes in middle ear mechanics.

In Figure 5–17, it can be seen that the probability of being able to observe a normal reflex is reduced to 50 percent when a conduc-

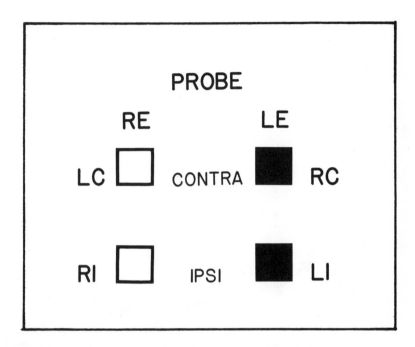

Figure 5–16. The vertical reflex pattern. Reflexes are abnormal with the probe in the left ear, independent of the location of the activator sound. This pattern represents a "probe effect."

tive component as small as 5 to 15 dB is present in the probe ear. In contrast, the same probability exists only when the conductive component exceeds 20 to 25 dB in the earphone ear. Thus, the attenuation factor produced by a middle ear disorder is more readily overcome than the mechanical disadvantage typical of that same disorder. When a vertical pattern appears, therefore, meticulous testing to rule out covert middle ear abnormality should be planned before attributing the reflex abnormality to facial nerve disorder or to an absent muscle.

The Unibox Pattern

This is a rare pattern, also unique to brain stem involvement. Here, only one crossed reflex (RC) is affected, whereas the other three remain normal (Fig. 5–18). We can deduce that there is no sound effect because the reflex is abnormal only on the RC configuration, rather than on both RC and RI. Similarly, there is no probe effect because a normal reflex appears with the probe in the right ear (RI and LC) as well as in the left ear (LI). Therefore, we cannot account

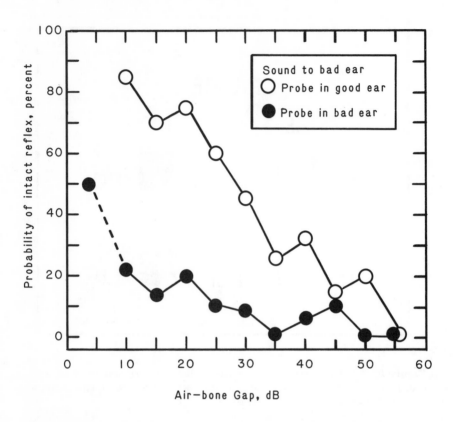

Figure 5-17. Probability of absent reflex as a function of air-bone gap when sound is directed to the affected ear (open circles) and when the probe is in the affected ear (closed circles).

for the pattern of disturbances in the afferent or efferent limbs of the reflex arc. A midline brain stem disorder in the region of the trapezoid body would affect both crossed reflexes, as in the horizontal pattern. The single abnormal reflex, therefore, reflects dysfunction confined to the region of a single superior olivary complex, in this case the left.

This pattern may appear with diseases producing scattered or discrete lesions in the brain stem, as may occur with multiple sclerosis. It can also represent the effect of a tumor occurring above the olivary nuclei that has extended caudally into a single area.

The Inverted-L Pattern

This pattern can be produced either peripherally or centrally.

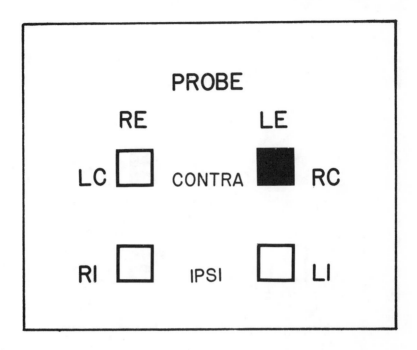

Figure 5–18. The uni-box reflex pattern. Reflexes are abnormal on one contralateral reflex only (RC).

Peripheral Source. The usual source of the inverted-L pattern on a peripheral basis is a unilateral middle ear disorder. Such a disorder has two effects on sound transmission. First, the impedance-matching function of the affected middle ear is made less effective; and second, as a result of the inefficient impedance match, the signal is attenuated before it arrives at the cochlea for the first stage of the reflex arc. Thus, there is both a probe effect that prevents observation of any reflex and a sound effect related to attenuation of the activator signal.

These effects are apparent in the example in Figure 5–19. When the activator is directed to the right ear through the probe (RI), a normal reflex can be observed. This indicates that both the afferent and the efferent systems are probably intact in the right ear. When the activator is directed to the left ear while the probe is in the healthy right ear (LC), the reflex is abnormal or absent. This reflects the attenuation produced by the middle ear problem on the left. For example, if a conductive hearing impairment of 40 dB is present at the test frequency, a sound of 110 dB delivered to the

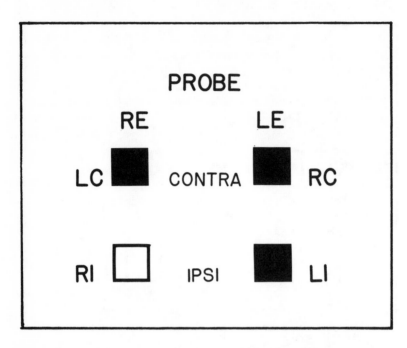

Figure 5–19. The inverted-L pattern. Reflexes are normal on one ipsilateral reflex only (RI). This pattern may be produced by either peripheral or retrocochlear disorders.

eardrum arrives at the cochlea with an intensity of only about 70 dB. For many individuals, that level is insufficient to cause an observable reflex. The same problem of attenuation occurs when the activator is presented to the left ear through the probe (LI). Additionally, the pathologic lesion responsible for the conductive hearing loss on the left prevents the probe from "seeing" the impedance change produced by a stapedial contraction. That is, the muscle contraction cannot alter acoustic impedance sufficiently to be recognized by the equipment. Hence, although stimulation of the healthy right ear may well generate a crossed (right-to-left) reflex (RC), the abnormally high or low impedance in the probe ear is not altered significantly by the muscle's contraction and the reflex appears to be "absent." This pattern therefore represents a pure sound effect on the LC, a pure probe effect on the RC, and a combined probe and sound effect on the LI.

Central Source. When an inverted-L pattern appears as a result of a retrocochlear disorder, it usually represents a combination of effects that, like the peripheral pattern, can be analyzed individually.

First, the inverted-L pattern often appears with a large acoustic tumor in the internal auditory canal. As we have established, eighth nerve disorders are characterized by a diagonal pattern. With continued enlargement of the tumor, the facial nerve (also located in the IAC) may become involved, causing a facial paralysis or weakness. That situation is reflected in a vertical pattern. Thus, a large tumor on the right would appear as a right diagonal plus a right vertical to yield the inverted-L pattern (Fig. 5–20). In this example, a pure sound effect and a pure probe effect coexist in the right ear; only the LI reflects normal function on the left. Of course, mild middle ear disorder on the right must be carefully excluded as a contributing factor.

Second, as shown in Figure 5–21, the inverted-L pattern may represent in part a horizontal pattern produced by a disorder in the brain stem. In this case, both crossed reflexes would be abnormal or absent. That pattern, combined with a diagonal pattern representing a severe hearing loss or a lesion of the right eighth nerve or cochlear nucleus, would combine to produce the inverted L.

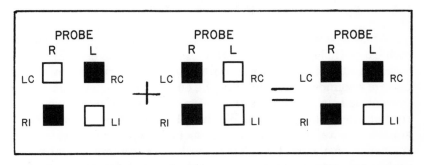

Figure 5–20. The retrocochlear inverted-L pattern is produced by a combination of a diagonal and a vertical pattern on the right.

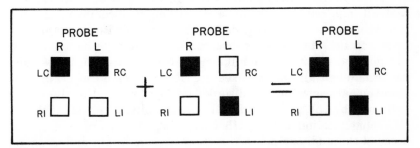

Figure 5–21. An inverted-L pattern produced by a combination of a horizontal and a diagonal pattern.

Similarly, a horizontal pattern may combine with a vertical pattern to produce the same results (Fig. 5–22).

Finally, as in Figure 5–23, the inverted L can occur when a unibox pattern is accompanied by either a diagonal or vertical pattern. These combinations are to be found in patients who have diffuse or widespread brain stem pathology.

The Four-Square Pattern

In this pattern (Fig. 5–24), all four reflexes are abnormal or absent. It may occur on either a peripheral or (more rarely) a central basis. When only peripheral dysfunction exists, the pattern suggests either a middle ear or a cochlear site. A bilateral middle ear disorder results in simultaneous sound and probe effects. That is, the activator sound is attenuated by the ineffective impedance mismatch in the middle ear; at the same time, the condition that has developed to produce the impedance mismatch will prevent measurement of any reflex that might occur if the attenuation factor can be overcome by the activator level. Abnormal tympanometry, static compliance, or a measurable air-bone gap on pure tone audiometry will help localize the source of this pattern to the middle ears.

When a severe to profound sensitivity loss exists as a result of cochlear pathology, the four-square pattern may also result. In this case, the absent or abnormal reflexes can be accounted for on the basis of a sound effect; generally, the output limits of our equipment prevent us from presenting the activator at a level high enough to compensate for the widespread hair cell loss (with or without degeneration of spiral ganglion fibers) responsible for such a severe hearing deficit. Although the effector mechanism (muscle, facial nerve, middle ear) may be intact bilaterally, the reflex fails because of an abnormality on the afferent limb of the arc.

Occasionally central auditory dysfunction may be so widespread that all four reflexes are affected. Although uncommon, acoustic tumors do occur bilaterally, usually in persons with neurofibromatosis (von Recklinghausen's disease). Brain stem pathology involving large areas of the medulla may also produce the four-square pattern. When all four reflexes are absent because of brain stem involvement, however, the disorder can be localized to the region delimited by the cochlear nuclei and the olivary nuclei. There is still some question as to whether pathologic lesions in more rostral areas of the auditory nervous system (i.e., midbrain and temporal cortex) exert an influence on characteristics of the acoustic reflex. Abnormalities in the form of low thresholds and very high ampli-

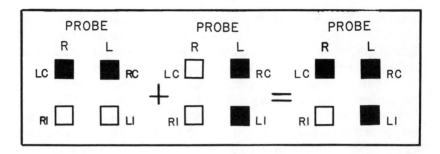

Figure 5–22. An inverted-L pattern produced by a combination of a horizontal and a vertical pattern.

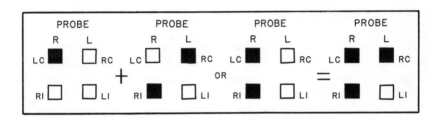

Figure 5–23. An inverted-L pattern produced by a combination of a unibox with a diagonal or vertical pattern.

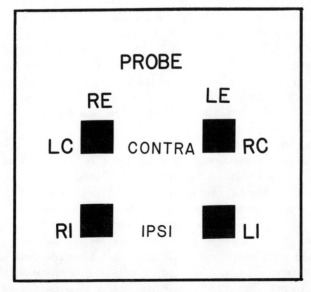

Figure 5–24. The four-square reflex pattern. All reflexes are abnormal.

tudes have been reported by some investigators (Downs and Crum, 1980; Jerger and Jerger, 1981), who view them as signs of the loss of central inhibitory influences on the reflex, although others (Gelfand and Silman, 1982) have challenged this interpretation.

The importance of interpreting acoustic reflex patterns within the context of a test battery cannot be overemphasized. These patterns can provide sensitive and reliable signs of auditory dysfunction at levels ranging from the middle ear to the brain stem; such signs, however, serve primarily as guidelines to the clinician for developing a precise and economical test battery for the remainder of the assessment.

CONCLUSIONS

The process of using immittance measurement as a guide to possible source of auditory dysfunction is based on the same philosophy that underlies medical diagnosis. For example, a patient decides to consult a physician about a skin rash. After eliciting details of his or her medical, social, and family history, the physician measures and records the patient's blood pressure, temperature, and pulse rate. The presence of a fever would suggest some bacterial infection; the physician will then evaluate the patient's rash while thinking about possible bacterial infections that are known to cause rashes. The visual appearance of the rash rules out a few possibilities and strengthens others; the history does the same. Further testing continues until a diagnosis is reached.

Similarly, immittance results let us construct a set of working hypotheses about the nature of a patient's auditory dysfunction very early in the evaluation and lead us to look for the appropriate cross-checks during each step of the remaining procedure. Table 5-1 summarizes the hypotheses that follow various combinations of immittance results.

Note first that when all three components of the battery—static compliance, tympanometry, and acoustic reflexes—are completely normal, we can assume two things: (1) There is not a total loss of hearing on either ear because sensitivity must be better than 80–85 dB HL to produce a reflex at all, and better than about 60 dB HL for reflexes to be present at a normal threshold; (2) there is no significant middle ear dysfunction. Therefore, any sensitivity loss later identified with pure tone audiometry can be accounted for by dysfunction in the cochlea or eighth nerve—a sensorineural impairment. Normal immittance results would also be expected when

Table 5-1. Summary of Hypotheses Based on Combined Immittance Results

Static Compliance	Tympanogram	Reflexes	Hypothesis
Normal[a]	Normal[b]	Normal[c]	Normal hearing or Sensorineural >60 dB HL or Central above SOC[d]
Abnormal or normal	Abnormal	Normal	Normal hearing or Mild conductive
Normal	Normal	Abnormal	Mild conductive or Sensorineural >60 dB HL or VIIIth nerve or Brain stem or VIIth nerve
Abnormal	Abnormal	Abnormal	Conductive or Mixed

a 0.3–1.6 cc
b Type A
c Ipsi/contra reflex threshold ≤ 100 dB HL, no decay
d Superior olivary complex

central auditory dysfunction exists above the brainstem because the reflex arc would not be affected by such a condition.

Second, a result in which acoustic reflexes appeared at normal thresholds even though static compliance or tympanometry were abnormal would suggest a mild middle ear disorder that does not attenuate the activator stimulus sufficiently to raise its threshold, and still permits monitoring of the small immittance changes caused by stapedial contraction. In such a case, only a slight conductive component (if any) of the total sensitivity loss would be expected.

Third is the case when both static compliance and tympanometry are normal but acoustic reflexes are abnormal in some way. The abnormalities, however, appear in *patterns* that can only be accounted for by a limited number of conditions. Therefore, the number of working hypotheses on which to base the rest of the evaluation are again restricted.

Refer to Table 5-2; you will see, for example, that the diagonal pattern is typical only of severe to profound cochlear impairment and of retrocochlear eighth nerve disorder, whereas the inverted-L pattern is compatible only with a conductive or retrocochlear dysfunction. In each case the basic distinction can be made once pure tone sensitivity is known and appropriate testing is then planned to support the impression.

Finally, when all three components of the battery are abnormal, there is strong evidence of middle ear dysfunction on one or both ears (again, depending on the reflex pattern) and therefore conductive components to any hearing impairment should be anticipated. It is wise to remember, however, that although measurement of acoustic immittance is most sensitive to middle ear disorders, such disorders can—and do—co-exist with more serious problems in the cochlea, auditory nerve, and central auditory nervous system.

At the beginning of this chapter it was noted that the information provided by immittance measures offers several advantages over conventional pure tone audiometry in the evaluation of auditory dysfunction. As you have probably realized by now, the use of the two procedures is actually *interdependent* rather than *independent*. That is, immittance measures validate and enrich the information contained in a pure tone audiogram, and the significance of immittance results becomes clear when they are related to the patient's pure tone sensitivity. Thus, pure tone audiometry will be the topic of Chapter 6.

STUDY QUESTIONS

Tympanometry and Static Compliance

1. Why is it important to complete an otoscopic examination before starting acoustic immittance measurements?

2. Is immittance a test of hearing? Why or why not?

3. What are the three components housed in the impedance probe tip and what are their purposes?

4. Explain the concept of an "equivalent volume" of the ear (i.e., why is the volume "equivalent" rather than "absolute"?).

Table 5-2. Patterns of Acoustic Reflex Abnormalities

SITE OF DISORDER	1	2	3	4	5	6	7	8
Middle ear			●				●	●
Cochlea	●	●						●
VIIIth nerve		●					●	
Brain stem (low)					●	●	●	●
Brain stem (high)	●					●		
Temporal lobe	●							

5. Why is a low frequency (220–226 Hz) probe tone more commonly used for tympanometry than one of a higher frequency?

6. At what point on the pressure-compliance is the canal SPL the lowest in a normal ear? Where would it be greatest?

7. What tympanometric features would allow you to distinguish between an open and occluded PE tube? Between an intact and a perforated tympanic membrane?

8. Why is static compliance considered the weakest measure of middle ear function in the immittance battery?

Acoustic Reflexes

1. What anatomical and physiological features must be present in order to observe a normal acoustic reflex?

2. Do normal acoustic reflexes indicate normal hearing sensitivity? Why or why not?

3. Differentiate between the probe effect and the sound effect in analyzing patterns of acoustic reflex abnormality.

4. Acoustic reflexes are often described as "absent" bilaterally when a middle ear disorder exists on only one ear. How can you qualify that statement to make it more accurate?

5. When measuring the contralateral acoustic reflex, is the "probe ear" or the "earphone ear" the one under test? Why?

6. A patient with unilateral facial paralysis, evaluated with immittance audiometry, shows normal acoustic reflexes on each ear. What level of facial nerve disorder could you infer from these results? Why?

7. How would collapsing ear canals produce a horizontal pattern of reflex abnormality?

Chapter 6

Pure Tone Audiometry

In the discussion of immittance audiometry, we learned that (1) the mechanical status of the middle ear can be evaluated using tympanometry and estimates of static compliance; and (2) a set of working hypotheses about possible sites of auditory disorder can be formulated by evaluating patterns of acoustic reflex abnormality. This information, however, is based on the efficiency with which a single, low frequency signal—the probe tone—is transmitted through a system under several mechanical conditions. Despite its many advantages, the results of immittance measures permit only inferences about a patient's auditory status, not direct answers. For example, abnormal tympanometry or acoustic reflexes suggest a middle ear disorder, which by definition produces a conductive hearing impairment. Immittance results provide no frequency-specific information, however, nor do they specify the severity of the impairment. More seriously, clues to the presence of a co-existing sensory or neural disorder are usually obscured by the more peripheral disorder when acoustic reflexes cannot be measured.

Pure tone audiometry supplements the information yielded by immittance audiometry in three major ways: First, it specifies how well a range of frequencies is transmitted through the entire peripheral auditory system, not just the middle ear. Second, the meaning of patterns of acoustic reflex abnormalities can be interpreted with greater precision once pure tone sensitivity is known. Third, several questions about an individual's auditory status can be answered:

- Is there evidence of a hearing impairment?
- If so, how severe is the impairment?
- Is the impairment conductive, sensorineural, or mixed?

Direct answers to these questions are sought in pure tone audiometry by making a series of comparisons. The question of the presence and magnitude of a sensitivity impairment is answered by comparing the subject's ability to hear tones of several frequencies to a set of standards that define the ranges of "normal" and impaired hearing. Comparison of sensitivity for air- and bone-conducted stimuli determines how much of a given sensitivity impairment can be accounted for by a middle ear disorder and how much by a sensorineural deficit.

If the descriptive information provided by pure tone audiometry is subjected to the same processes of logical deduction used to analyze patterns of acoustic reflex abnormality, patterns of pure tone abnormality also emerge that allow us to go beyond the "what" and "how much" of hearing impairment and to approach the question of "why." Ideally, the accounts developed for abnormal immittance results and for abnormal pure tone results will support each other, satisfying the cross-check principle. If the accounts do not support each other, the inconsistencies must be accounted for by recognizing sources of error in the test technique or environment, subject, or tester.

The following sections will present the principles of measuring and interpreting sensitivity for air- and bone-conducted pure tones, principles of masking, relationships of pure tone to immittance results, and sources of error in pure tone audiometry.

THE MEANING OF "THRESHOLD"

In its earliest usage, *threshold* referred to a wooden bar or stone in the floor of a doorway, marking the passage into a house or room. Later, the term came to be used in a more general sense, suggesting the beginning of an experience or a state, and was symbolized by the practice of carrying a bride over the threshold of her new home. Only recently has "threshold" been used in the context of psychophysical measurements to describe the lowest intensity at which a given stimulus can elicit a specified response. Thresholds of auditory detection, discomfort, acoustic reflexes, speech reception, and speech detection (to name a few) represent different aspects of auditory function and are determined for various reasons in the clinical assessment of hearing.

Pure tone audiometry is based on establishing auditory detection thresholds in decibels for tones as a function of frequency. The measurement of such thresholds is approached with one of two goals in mind.

One goal is to define the best possible sensitivity of the human ear—an "absolute" threshold. This information is typically sought by psychoacousticians using very precise instruments to present small increments of perfectly controlled stimuli, over hundreds of trials, to highly trained listeners in virtually noise-free environments. The thresholds thus obtained relate only to the physical properties of the stimulus and their effects on perception, not to the expected or observed responses of any other listeners. The other goal—that sought in the clinic—is to define a subject's "relative" thresholds. In this case, the stimuli are usually presented in large (5 dB) steps to an untrained subject over relatively few trials in a reduced noise (but not "soundproofed") room. The subject's auditory sensitivity is then compared to the modal sensitivity of thousands of "normal" listeners who have been presented with the same stimuli. Thus, an absolute threshold gives direct information about an individual listener's sensitivity to stimuli of known dimensions; a relative threshold gives information about a listener's sensitivity compared to a norm. It is important to recognize this distinction and to understand that clinical "threshold" estimation represents only an approximation and not a direct indication of physiological state. There is no more succinct illustration of this difference than that provided by the changing standard for audiometric zero. As the norms have changed, so have the criteria for "normal" and "impaired" hearing.

"Relative" threshold and its associated unit of measurement, audiometric zero, forms the basis for the clinical evaluation of pure tone sensitivity. Remember that a decibel is based on the logarithm of a ratio between a reference and an output sound. The reference value must be specified to give meaning to the output. When sound pressure level (SPL) is used, the reference is 20 micropascals (μPa). Sound pressure levels can also be referred to 0.0002 dyne/cm^2, to 0.0002 microbar, and to 2×12^{-5} Newtons/m^2. Whatever the terminology used, 0 dB means only that the output level is exactly the same as the reference level, as in the following examples:

$$dB\ SPL = 20\ \log P_o\ /\ P_r$$

$$dB\ SPL = 20\ \log 0.0002/0.0002 \qquad dB\ SPL = 20\ \log 20/20$$
$$dB\ SPL = 20\ \log 1 \qquad dB\ SPL = 20\ \log 1$$
$$\log 1 = 0 \qquad \log 1 = 0$$
$$dB\ SPL = 20 \times 0 = 0 \qquad dB\ SPL = 20 \times 0 = 0$$

In these examples, 0 dB SPL, whether measured in Pascals, dynes, microbars, or Newtons, would express an equivalent pressure or force per unit area. However, if we wanted to express sound intensity relative to the average level on a freeway (FW) at rush hour (say, 80 dB SPL), 0 dB would have quite a different implication insofar as its absolute signal magnitude is concerned:

$$dB\ FW = 20\ \log 80/80$$
$$dB\ FW = 20\ \log 1$$
$$dB\ FW = 0$$

In this example, "0 dB FW" would be 10,000 times greater than 0 dB SPL! Therefore, if hearing sensitivity is to be measured in decibels, it is essential to note its reference value. If the reference value changes, the meaning of the output level changes as well.

The minimum audible pressure or equal loudness curve presented in Figure 6–1 shows the way in which sensitivity of the human ear varies with frequency. Each point represents the sound pressure level at the eardrum (MAP) needed to produce the same minimum level of audibility in normal human listeners. It is not always possible, however, to measure the SPL at the eardrum; for that reason, minimum audible pressure curves were described for sound pressure delivered through a specified coupler and measured at the meatus of the external auditory canal (MAPC). This curve is superimposed on the MAP curves in Figure 6–1. Differences in the two curves can be accounted for mainly by loss of the canal resonance. Notice that in each curve, higher sound pressure level is required for the beginning perception of low frequency sounds than for mid- and high-frequency sounds. Because the MAPC curve represents a standard of "normal" sensitivity, the sound pressure levels necessary for minimum audibility are used as the reference (P_r in the decibel equation) or baseline against which the sensitivity of clinical subjects can be compared at each frequency. That reference sound pressure level is represented by 0 on the audiometer dial (audiometric zero). Table 6–1 shows the norms for audiometric zero established by the American National Standards Institute (ANSI) in 1969.

If a subject's detection threshold in dB SPL at a given frequency is equal to the standard for audiometric zero at that frequency, his

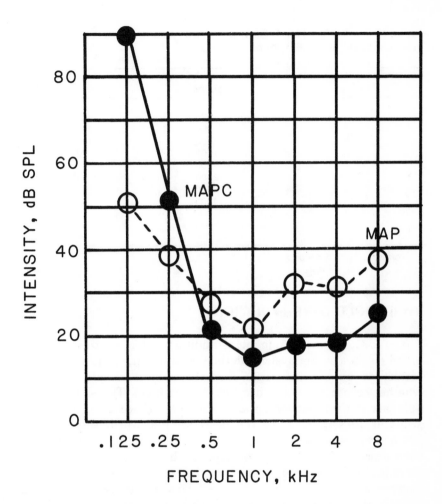

Figure 6–1. Minimum audible pressure (MAP) curves, demonstrating the way in which sensitivity of the ear varies with frequency. Note that greater sound pressure levels are needed at low and high frequencies than for mid-frequency sounds to produce the same minimum level of audibility.

or her threshold is recorded as 0 dB HL (hearing level). If, on the other hand, more (or less) sound pressure is needed by a subject to detect a pure tone, the threshold is higher (or lower) than 0. Like "relative pressure" in tympanometry, audiometric zero is used to express hearing sensitivity relative to a specified standard, the value of which is subject to change.

Table 6-1. ANSI (1969) Standards for Audiometric Zero: Sound Pressure Level at the Earphone

When the Audiometer Dial Reads	And the Frequency Is	The Actual SPL* Is
0	125	45.0
0	250	25.5
0	500	11.5
0	1000	7.0
0	1500	6.5
0	2000	9.0
0	3000	10.0
0	4000	9.5
0	6000	15.5
0	8000	13.0

*Norms for TDH-39 earphones

THRESHOLD DETERMINATION

The traditional measurement of auditory detection thresholds is based on the psychophysical Method of Limits (i.e., the stimulus is controlled by the examiner and the subject simply indicates whether or not he or she has heard the sound). Threshold can be approached using either an *ascending* or a *descending* method of stimulus presentation. In the descending method, the test run begins at a level estimated to be clearly audible to the subject and then descends until he or she reports that the tone is no longer audible. In the ascending method, the test tone is presented initially at a very low intensity (e.g., −10 dB) and is then raised until the subject signals that he or she has detected it. The majority of audiology clinics use the Hughson-Westlake modification of the ascending method (Carhart and Jerger, 1959). In this method, the signal is first presented at a clearly audible level and then is lowered in 10 dB steps until it becomes inaudible. At this point, the signal level is increased in 5 dB steps until the patient once again begins to respond. Each time a response occurs the signal level is reduced and the next ascending series of stimulus presentations begins. Threshold is recorded as that intensity level at which the subject responds correctly to 50 percent or more of the signal presentations. Examples of threshold approximations using the three methods are shown in Figure 6-2.

It is important to note that the level recorded as a subject's threshold after this type of measurement procedure may not corres-

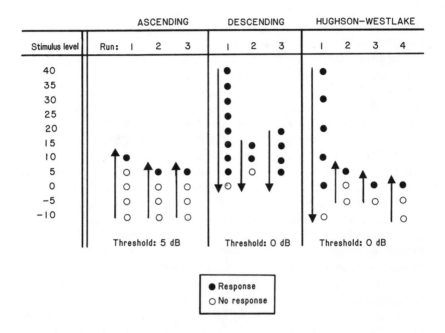

Figure 6–2. Pure tone threshold approximations produced by ascending, descending, and Hughson-Westlake stimulus presentation methods.

pond to his or her absolute threshold, usually defined as the level at which a listener is able to identify a signal correctly 50 percent of the time. The clinical practice of establishing relative thresholds using increments of 5 dB was designed to provide an efficient first approximation of hearing, not to define absolute threshold. Therefore, a subject whose "true" threshold was 7 dB HL would not respond to a tone presented at 5 dB but would respond to a 10 dB presentation more than 50 percent of the time.

When greater precision in threshold estimation is demanded, techniques other than the method of limits should be used. *Adaptive procedures* are used in most psychoacoustic laboratories and offer greater flexibility in step size, thus allowing more narrow estimates of threshold. In addition, modifications of the adaptive procedures allow estimation of values other than 50 percent on the psychometric function, such as 25 or 75 percent response. Because adaptive techniques use rules for raising or lowering stimulus levels based on how the subject responded to the previous stimuli, they are easily programmed for use in a computer-based audiometer. Although such techniques are usually unnecessary for the usual clinical diagnostic application, they are finding more use in assessing progress to criterion performance in aural rehabilitation programs or in hearing aid selection procedures.

Auditory detection thresholds are determined for a range of frequencies, encompassing the range from 250 to 8000 Hz in octave intervals (250, 500, 1000 Hz, etc.) and are recorded on an audiogram (Fig. 6–3). By convention, frequencies are represented at octave (and some midoctave) intervals along the abscissa and signal intensity in dB HL along the ordinate, with 0 dB toward the top of the audiogram. The axes should be clearly labeled, with the reference standard (ISO, ANSI, etc.) noted. The audiogram presents threshold information about a listener's sensitivity for pure tones presented by air conduction and bone conduction. It is convenient to record acoustic reflex thresholds on the same grid to allow direct comparison of detection and reflex thresholds. Once thresholds have been established, the audiogram is classified with respect to (1) the magnitude or severity of any impairment noted; and (2) the configuration of the impairment. The type of hearing impairment—conductive, sensorineural, or mixed—cannot be established on the basis of air conduction thresholds alone. Therefore, we turn now to a consideration of the two modes of sound transmission—air conduction and bone conduction.

MODES OF SOUND TRANSMISSION

Air Conduction

Students who have completed coursework in auditory anatomy and physiology have studied the mechanisms of air conduction in some detail. Therefore, this section is purposely brief and will not attempt to reiterate the principles covered in such courses, but instead will consider the mechanisms of bone conduction in greater detail. Excellent discussions of air conduction are available; several sources are listed in the suggested readings at the end of the book.

Sound is said to be air-conducted when it is transmitted through the (normally) air-filled external ear canal and middle ear space to the cochlea. This is the usual way in which we receive sound from the environment; therefore, measuring sensitivity to air-conducted sounds has some immediate practical significance. Air conduction thresholds represent the cumulative efficiency with which sound is conducted through outer, middle, and inner ear structures. Elevated air conduction thresholds, therefore, may appear as a consequence

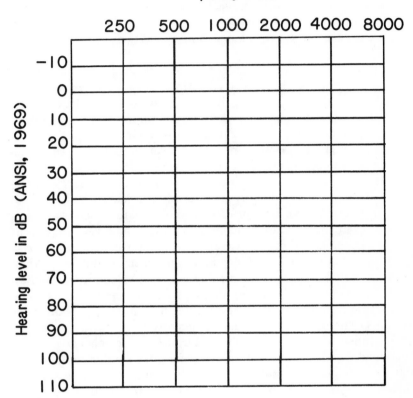

Figure 6–3. An audiogram used to present pure tone sensitivity data. Frequency in kHz is on the abscissa; intensity in dB HL is on the ordinate.

of blockage in the ear canal, of impedance mismatches in the middle ear structures, of damaged or missing sensory or neural elements in the inner ear, or of any combination of those circumstances. As a result, air conduction is a nonspecific measure that must be supplemented by other procedures to define the nature of the impairment. Immittance audiometry provides general information about outer and middle ear status; bone conduction audiometry provides frequency-specific information about sensorineural status.

Bone Conduction

Most people, on hearing their own tape-recorded voices for the first time, are shocked at its unfamiliar quality. We hear the tape-recorded signal as it is transmitted by air conduction alone, which is the mode in which others receive our speech. However, our own vocalizations travel to the cochlea by both air and bone conduction; this is the basis for the usual objection, "That doesn't sound like me at all!"

If you hold your finger against the side of your nose while humming, you can feel the bones vibrating; the vibrations are more noticeable with a low-pitched hum than when the voice is high-pitched. In this example, the vibrating air column travels and resonates along the vocal tract, causing direct vibration of the skull bones in the process. Bone conduction of sound results in the same hydromechanical and electrochemical events in the cochlea as those produced by air conduction; mechanical transfer of energy to the cochlea from the sound source, however, is accomplished by skull vibration rather than by vibration of the tympanic membrane and ossicles exclusively. This principle has proved to be very important in the assessment of conductive hearing impairments, which arise because of inefficient impedance matching in the middle ear. When such a condition exists, bone conduction thresholds are lower than air conduction thresholds because the latter represent, as mentioned, the cumulative efficiency of the outer, middle, and inner ear systems, whereas bone conduction sensitivity is most representative of inner ear status only. The difference in decibels between the threshold for air conduction and that for bone conduction is called the *air-bone gap*. The notion that bone conduction "bypasses" the middle ear structures in transmitting sound to the inner ear, however, is not completely accurate, as the following discussion will illustrate.

Purpose of Bone Conduction Measurement

Air conduction thresholds, like many other tests used in the audiometric battery, provide information that can be used in more than one way—for example, for purposes of diagnosis, predicting hearing aid gain, and monitoring treatment efficacy. Bone conduction thresholds, however, are used only for comparison with air conduction thresholds, to determine whether a hearing impairment is conductive, sensorineural, or mixed. Detailed criteria for classification of audiograms based on air and bone conduction thresholds are presented in a later section.

Mechanisms of Bone Conduction

Think of the ossicular chain suspended by ligaments within the temporal bone. When the skull vibrates as a unit, the inertia of the ossicles causes their motion to lag behind that of the skull, because they are not rigidly attached to it. Thus, the stapes moves out of phase with the oval window, causing a disturbance of the cochlear fluids. This process is called *inertial bone conduction*. Because the skull vibrates as a unit only for frequencies of 800 Hz or lower, inertial bone conduction makes its greatest contribution to the transmission of low frequency signals.

When higher frequency vibrations are applied to the skull, it vibrates segmentally. That is, opposite areas of the skull may move out of phase with each other. The effect of these opposing forces is that the bony walls of the cochlea are periodically deformed, compressing the channels containing the cochlear fluids. As a result, fluid pressure changes within the cochlea are relieved by movement of the membranes covering the oval and round windows. As the round window membrane bulges out into the middle ear space, the stapes is drawn into the oval window; thus, the two windows (and the stapes) move 180 degrees out of phase with each other. Just as in the case of air conduction, a traveling wave is set up on the basilar membrane by the fluid pressure changes, and, as a result, the stereocilia of the hair cells are deformed against the tectorial membrane. This process is called *compressional bone conduction*. Notice again that the middle ear does participate in this type of bone conduction.

A third mechanism in which bone conduction transmission occurs was described by Tonndorf (1966, 1972). When the skull vibrates, some energy is radiated into the external ear canal, creating sound waves that may travel through the usual air conduction pathways of the middle ear. Under ordinary circumstances the ear canal acts as a high pass (low cut) filter; if it is closed off (occluded) while the skull is vibrating, more low frequency sound is trapped in the canal and transferred to the tympanic membrane. Therefore, the total amount of sound energy arriving at the cochlea would be greater when the ear canal is occluded, because there are contributions by both bone conduction and air conduction. This is called the *occlusion effect*, and it is easily demonstrated by plugging one ear with your finger as you talk. The magnitude of the effect is calculated by subtracting bone conduction thresholds determined while the ear is occluded from those determined in an unoccluded condition. In subjects with normal middle ear mechanisms, the occlusion effect varies from more than 20 dB at 250 Hz to 0 dB at frequencies of 2000 Hz and higher, as illustrated in Figure 6-4. Subjects with middle ear disorders, however, show little or no effect of occlusion on bone conduction thresholds, probably because the efficiency of the

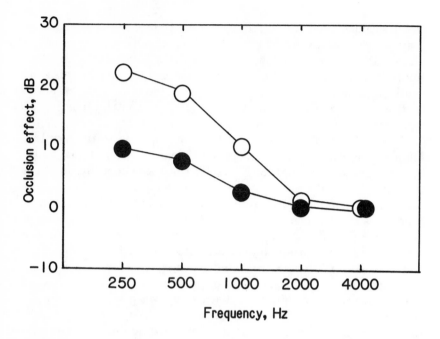

Figure 6–4. Magnitude of the occlusion effect as a function of frequency. Note that the largest effect is in the low frequencies. Earphones enclosing a larger volume (Sharpe HA-10) have a smaller occlusion effect. Modified from Hodgson, W., and Tillman, T. (1966).

air conduction system has been reduced by the loss of effective impedance matching in the middle ear. Measurement of the occlusion effect (referred to as the *occlusion index*) offers an important cross-check in the assessment of conductive impairments; an occlusion index lower than the norm for the test frequency—usually 500 Hz—supports the impression of a conductive disorder, whereas large occluded-unoccluded threshold differences suggest normal middle ear function.

Theoretically, sensitivity to bone conducted signals can be no worse than that for an air conducted signal because the cochlea is the peripheral endpoint for both routes. In practice, however, the many sources of variance in testing bone conduction (see Chapter 9) may produce results that are more heavily influenced by measurement procedures than by physiological status. For this reason, careful use of the appropriate cross-checks is always wise.

Interaural Attenuation

One of the most important principles to remember about bone conduction is that *vibration of the skull affects both cochleas equally and simultaneously.* This means that a vibratory force applied to the right side of the head is able to stimulate both the right and the left cochlea and is sometimes referred to as "cross-over." Another way of saying this is that there is 0 dB *interaural attenuation* during bone conduction; that is, essentially no sound energy is lost in radiating to all portions of the skull.

Bone conduction can be produced in two ways, directly and indirectly. In the direct mode, a vibrating transducer, the bone oscillator, is applied to the head and, as already explained, stimulates both cochleas equally and simultaneously. In the indirect mode, the output sound pressure level of the speaker encased in the earphone is sufficient to cause vibration not only of the air molecules trapped between the speaker and the tympanic membrane but also of the skull bones, once their greater impedance is overcome. Air conducted stimulus intensities in the range of 40 to 60 dB HL are sufficient to cause cross-over in most persons. That is, a 40 to 60 dB interaural attenuation exists for air conducted stimuli. Once the stimulus is being delivered—even in part—by bone conduction, however, both ears can respond. Thus, the practical significance of interaural attenuation lies in specifying to what extent one ear can be tested independently of the other; in the case of air conduction, cross-over of the test signal does not occur until its signal intensity exceeds 40 to 60 dB, providing some isolation of the test and nontest ears. For bone conduction, in which interaural attenuation is essentially 0 dB, the ears cannot be tested independently unless the threshold of the nontest ear can be raised. This is accomplished by means of a process called *masking,* and will be considered in detail in Chapter 7.

THE STENGER TEST

Asymmetry in auditory function should always be a "red flag" to the clinician and prompt detailed investigation into the nature of the disorder. Most often, asymmetrical or unilateral impairment is produced by a significant pathologic condition limited to one ear. Such impairment, however, can also occur on a nonorganic basis, either intentionally as in malingering, or as a psychogenic overlay to an organically based problem. The Stenger test is a procedure that can be used conveniently during pure tone audiometry to verify asymmetries in voluntary pure tone thresholds.

Most of us have experienced the unique sensation of listening to music through earphones; the music seems to fill the center of the head, rather than being confined to the two ears. If one channel were attenuated, however, the midline image would be lost and the music would seem to be located at the ear in which it was loudest.

This phenomenon, called the *Stenger effect,* forms the basis for a simple and effective test used to validate interaural threshold differences. The test can be administered using either pure tones or speech as stimuli and should be a part of the test battery whenever a threshold difference of 15 dB or more exists between the two ears. Even if there is evidence from the history or immittance results that could account for threshold asymmetry, the Stenger test should be administered to rule out the contribution of a "functional" (nonorganic) overlay to the impairment.

The pure tone Stenger test requires that tones of identical frequency and phase be presented simultaneously through earphones. The patient is instructed to raise the hand corresponding to the ear in which the tone is heard, to keep this hand raised for the duration of the tone, and to lower or change hands if the tone disappears or changes location, respectively.

The test tone is introduced into both ears at a level 10 dB higher than the threshold of the "good" or control ear (10 dB SL). At this level the tone should be audible 100 percent of the time—until the tone in the "bad" (test) ear achieves or exceeds the same loudness. At that point, the patient will either admit to the changing lateralization or will stop responding to the signal in the control ear. The following examples will illustrate how the test works.

Figure 6–5 shows the air conduction and acoustic reflex thresholds for both ears of a hypothetical patient. The left ear, with normal sensitivity, is the control ear; the right ear, with an average 55 dB impairment, is the test ear. Note first that acoustic reflex thresholds are within normal limits bilaterally. This result tells us (1) that the patient does not have a severe to profound loss in the right ear; and (2) that a middle ear disorder does not account for the impairment. The presence of normal reflexes, however, does not provide any specific information about peripheral hearing sensitivity, because normal reflex thresholds (≤ 100 dB HL) are maintained with impairments up to 60 to 65 dB HL.

For the Stenger test a 1000 Hz tone is presented to both ears simultaneously at 20 dB HL (10 dB SL reference: 1000 Hz threshold on the left). The patient raises his left hand without hesitation. The tone is then gradually withdrawn from the left ear, leaving it present in the right ear. The patient lowers his hand. The tone is

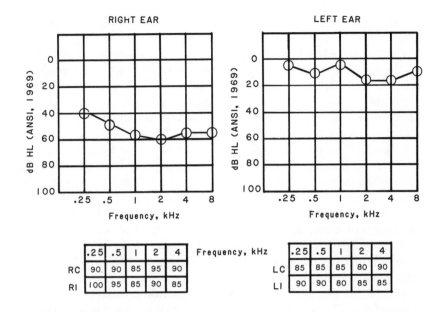

Figure 6–5. Audiometric data for a patient with an asymmetrical hearing impairment. A conductive basis for the loss is ruled out by the normal immittance results, but there is still a question as to the validity of the thresholds in the right ear.

returned to its original level in the left ear, and raised by 10 dB in the right ear; once again the patient responds to the control tone when it is present and stops responding when it is withdrawn. This process is repeated until the level of the test tone reaches 60 dB. At that point the patient begins to indicate some confusion, gesturing vaguely toward his head. A further 10 dB increment of the test tone brings an immediate elevation of the right hand, indicating that he hears the tone only in the right ear. At this point, the tone is withdrawn from the right ear, lateralizing the response back to the left ear. The test result is described as a negative Stenger, verifying the voluntary pure tone threshold at 1000 Hz on the right.

What are the dynamics of this sequence of behaviors? First, we can infer from the patient's immediate and positive lateralized response that the tone was audible in the control ear but not in the test ear. Second, the confusion that the patient manifested was evidence that the tones at the two ears were reaching equal loudness and a midline perception was beginning. Note that (at that point) the level of the test tone was only 5 dB SL reference: threshold in the right ear, whereas it was present at 10 dB SL in the control ear.

This amount of disparity between the two ears could be interpreted as a sign of recruitment in the right ear, an inference supported by the acoustic reflex thresholds. That is, loudness grew more rapidly in the right ear than in the left once threshold was exceeded. Third, the patient readily signaled the change in location of the tones at the appropriate levels. The clinician can proceed with the evaluation, having collected evidence against the contribution of a nonorganic component.

Now consider the same initial audiometric results as they relate to a second set of responses to the Stenger procedure. The 1000 Hz tone is delivered at 20 dB HL to both ears and the patient indicates that he hears the sound on the left. The control tone is withdrawn and the patient stops responding. On the next trial the control tone is present at 20 dB and the test tone at 30 dB. There is no response. When the tone is withdrawn from the test (right) ear, the patient once again responds appropriately to the tone in the left ear. The test tone is reintroduced and the patient stops responding. The result of this test is said to be positive by inhibition. So long as the tone was louder in the control ear, the patient responded willingly. Once the loudness of the tone was greater in the test ear, however, he became unaware of its presence in the control ear and, not wishing to acknowledge a low intensity signal in his allegedly impaired ear, stopped responding. If the voluntary threshold of 55 dB HL on the right was accurate, the response from the left ear could not have been suppressed as it was. Thus, this test result suggests a nonorganic auditory component with true sensitivity no worse than about 20 to 25 dB HL. Later in the evaluation, speech thresholds can be determined to cross-check that estimate.

A shorter version of the Stenger test can be administered by keeping the tone constant at 10 dB SL in the control ear and slowly increasing the intensity (ideally, by 1 to 2 dB steps) in the test ear. The patient is instructed to listen to the tone present in the "good" ear and to notify the clinician when the tone seems to begin moving toward the center of the head. In this way, the patient's attention is focused on the ear he or she has acknowledged as normal instead of having his or her cooperation challenged by focusing on the "bad" ear; the patient can, after all, simply refuse to continue with the test at any time. When the patient reports that the tone's location is starting to move out of the ear and into the head, it can be assumed that the loudness at the two ears is becoming equal and sensitivity can be approximated within about 10 dB.

Successful administration and interpretation of the Stenger test requires that the patient have essentially normal sensitivity in one ear. In addition, the audiometric equipment must have several features, most of which are standard on today's clinical audiometers. First, the audiometer must have *independent attenuators* for each channel, although separate oscillators are not necessary. Second, if separate oscillators are used, there must be some provision for *phase-locking the signals*; phase-locking is done automatically on audiometers that have a single oscillator and two attenuators because the identical signal is sent from the oscillator into the attenuators. Third, the *earphones must be phase-matched* so that the diaphragm of the earphone speakers will produce the same condensation or rarefaction impulse in the ear canal. Fourth, the *output SPL of the earphones must be equal* for the same attenuator dial reading, or the appropriate corrections must be applied before the tones are presented. Fifth, both *earphones must be activated simultaneously*, again to preserve the phase relationships of the signals at the two ears. Precise phase alignment is crucial to generate the maximum effect. Binaural tones that are presented out of phase, with unequal intensity, or with different onset-offset times allow the listener to perceive the tone in each ear rather than forming a midline or intracranial image.

STUDY QUESTIONS

1. What information does pure tone audiometry provide that is not given by immittance audiometry?

2. Distinguish between absolute and relative measures of threshold.

3. What is meant by audiometric zero?

4. Is audiometric zero based on MAP or MAPC data?

5. What is an audiogram?

6. What site of auditory disorder can be inferred from air conduction thresholds?

7. What is the purpose of measuring bone conduction thresholds?

8. How does inertial bone conduction take place?

9. Do bone conduction measurements bypass the middle ear and stimulate the cochlea directly? Explain your answer.

10. What is the occlusion effect?

11. Why is a low frequency signal used to calculate the occlusion index?

12. How does interaural attenuation occur?

13. Explain why interaural attenuation is greater for air conducted than for bone conducted signals.

14. What is the fallacy in doing unmasked bone conduction thresholds for each ear?

15. Why would an air-bone gap be present with conductive hearing impairment but not with sensorineural impairment?

16. If a patient had a total unilateral impairment (anacusis) would he respond to the signal if it were present at 75 dB HL in the test ear and 10 dB HL in the control ear? What would his response be if the tone were withdrawn from the control ear? Explain your answer.

Chapter 7

Principles of Masking

Masking is a part of our daily lives. It occurs when we try to have a quiet conversation in a noisy restaurant; when we fail to hear a doorbell or telephone ring while in the shower; while using a hairdryer. The common feature of these experiences is that some noise prevents us from hearing other sounds at their normal levels—that is, it raises our threshold. Although its effects can be inconvenient in our daily lives, masking is an essential tool in auditory assessment.

Three issues about masking govern its effective use in the clinical assessment of hearing: first, the conditions under which masking should be used; second, the type of sound to use as a masker; and third, masker levels necessary to isolate the test and nontest ears effectively.

WHEN TO USE MASKING

We have already established that an oscillating force applied directly to the head causes a simultaneous disturbance of both cochleas ("cross-over"). If the goal is to evaluate each ear separately, the first rule for when to use masking is

Use masking when testing bone conduction
and the air-bone gap is 10 dB or more.

When air conduction thresholds are symmetrical and the unmasked bone conduction threshold falls within 10 dB of the air conduction (i.e., the air-bone gap is less than 10 dB), masking is usually unnecessary. The unmasked bone conduction response is nonspecific, representing only the sensitivity of the *better* cochlea; for this reason, recording unmasked bone conduction thresholds for each ear represents at best a redundant effort and, at worst, a poor understanding of the underlying principles of bone conduction. When air conduction sensitivity is bilaterally symmetrical and bone conduction is equivalent to the air conduction thresholds, it can be inferred that neither ear has a larger air-bone gap than is evident with the unmasked bone conduction.

Masking is often required during air conduction testing as well. In contrast to direct skull vibration by application of a bone conduction oscillator, in which case the interaural attenuation is essentially zero, the IA for air conduction is on the order of 40 to 60 dB. This means that sound delivered to one ear will also be present in the other ear, but at a level some 40 to 60 dB lower. The nontest ear receives sounds by air conduction by way of acoustic leakage from the earphones as well as by bone conduction caused by high sound pressure levels generated against the head by the earphones. The amount of interaural attenuation present for an air conducted signal varies within that range, depending on the subject's head size and skull density, the type of earphones used and their position, and the signal frequency. Therefore, for purposes of deciding whether to use masking during air conduction measurements, the lowest amount of interaural attenuation—40 dB—is assumed. It may well be the case that the true value for a given subject is 47 or 58 or 52 dB, but serious errors can be avoided by adopting a conservative criterion:

> *Use masking when the signal intensity is*
> *40 dB higher than the bone conduction*
> *threshold in the nontest ear.*

Please note that the rule does *not* state that masking is used when the air conduction thresholds of the two ears differ by 40 dB or more. Rather, the 40 dB criterion difference is between the *air conduction threshold of the test ear* and the *bone conduction threshold of the nontest ear.* What is the basis for this rule? Cross-over occurs during air conduction testing when the intensity of the signals being delivered through the earphones is sufficient to cause vibration of the bones of the skull; sound is then received simultaneously in both cochleas. Therefore, two factors determine whether cross-

hearing occurs: the signal intensity (i.e., its ability to cause skull vibration) and the bone conduction sensitivity of the nontest ear (i.e., its ability to detect the skull vibrations).

A reasonable estimate of bone conduction sensitivity can be made by considering the results of the acoustic immittance testing that preceded pure tone audiometry. If the results of the immittance battery were completely normal, it can be safely assumed that there is no significant middle ear disorder. If there is no significant middle ear disorder, there is no air-bone gap; that is, air and bone conduction thresholds are the same. On the other hand, if the tympanogram or reflex pattern suggested a middle ear disorder, you must assume that an air-bone gap is present and that the bone conduction threshold is 0 dB. The data presented in Figure 7-1 can be used to illustrate this decision-making process.

Two identical air conduction audiograms appear in the right and left panels. At 1000 Hz, the right ear (RE) has a threshold of 30 dB HL and the left ear (LE) a threshold of 60 dB. Is masking required to rule out cross-hearing from the right ear? In panel A, note that static compliance and tympanometry were normal and that ipsilateral and contralateral acoustic reflexes were elicited at normal thresholds and with no adaptation. These results are indicative of normal middle ear function on the right; therefore, bone conduction and air conduction thresholds on the right ear are assumed to be the same—30 dB HL. Because the difference between the air conduction signal intensity in the left ear (60 dB) and the bone conduction threshold in the right ear (30 dB) does not differ by 40 dB or more, masking is not necessary at 1000 Hz. Now look at panel B. In this instance, abnormal immittance results were obtained on the right ear: very low static compliance, Type B tympanogram, and absent acoustic reflexes. A middle ear disorder is strongly indicated, and an air-bone gap would be predicted. In this case, the bone conduction threshold on the right ear is assumed to be 0 dB; again, the actual threshold may be higher or lower than 0, but we assume sensitivity equal to the standard, and that is 0 dB. Now the difference between the air conduction signal intensity in the left ear (60 dB) and the (assumed) bone conduction threshold in the right ear is 60 dB. Masking is necessary at that frequency to prove that the air conduction threshold on the left truly represents a response from the left ear, not cross-hearing from the right.

TYPES OF MASKING NOISE

The decision to use masking is made by recognizing the likelihood of cross-hearing under any given test condition. The next decision—

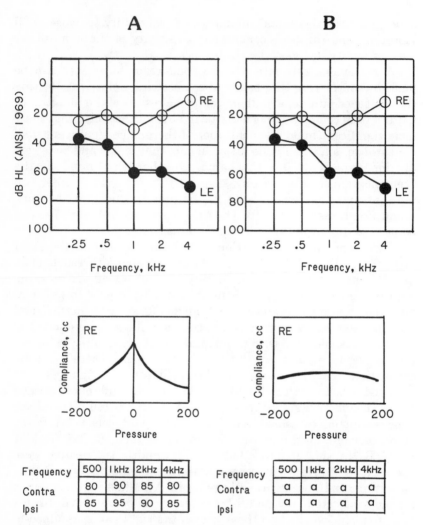

Figure 7-1. Audiometric data requiring a decision as to the necessity for masking during air conduction threshold measurement on the left. In Panel A, evidence of normal middle ear function is provided by the immittance results on the right; this suggests that bone conduction is no better than air conduction and therefore the interaural difference is not large enough to result in cross-hearing. In Panel B, there is evidence of a middle ear disorder on the right; therefore, cross-hearing is possible via bone conduction and masking would be required.

what kind of sound to use as a masker—is made by comparing the effectiveness and the efficiency of different kinds of noise. These characteristics are based on the concept of the critical band in masking.

When a test tone is presented in a broad band of noise, only a restricted band of frequencies centered on the frequency of the test tone acts to mask it. Frequencies higher or lower than those in the critical band can be removed without lessening the masking effect. The width of the critical band varies directly with frequency, as shown in Table 7–1.

Masking effectiveness (i.e., the ability to elevate threshold for a test tone) is determined by the acoustic energy present within the critical band. If the band is made more narrow, its masking effectiveness will be decreased unless the intensity of the smaller band is increased. If frequencies outside the critical band are added, masking effectiveness will not be affected, but masking efficiency will be reduced. This is because extra acoustic energy has been added to the noise, which does not increase its masking effectiveness. The optimum masker is the one that is most efficient—that is, the one that produces the most effective masking with the lowest overall intensity. Therefore, in determining which of several noises is the most efficient masker, we must consider its intensity within the critical band, not its overall SPL. The intensity of each frequency component of a band of noise is called its spectrum level (dB No) and is found by subtracting 10 times the log of the bandwidth from the total sound pressure level:

$$dB\ No = Total\ SPL - 10\ log\ bandwidth$$

Psychophysical experiments have shown that the most efficient masker is another tone identical or very close in frequency to that of the test tone. The spectrum level of a pure tone masker is the same as its overall sound pressure level because all of its acoustic energy is concentrated in one frequency, just as in the test tone. So, for a total SPL of 60 dB,

$$dB\ No = 60 - 10\ log\ 1$$
$$log\ 1 = 0$$
$$dB\ No = 60 - 0$$

Masking efficiency notwithstanding, tones are generally not used as maskers clinically because they would introduce confusion (for both patient and clinician) about which is test tone and which is masker. Instead, a noise composed of a broad spectrum of frequencies is used.

Two types of noises are commonly used as maskers in hearing assessment: broad band noise (BBN) and narrow band noise (NBN). Broad band noise has energy distributed at approximately equal amplitude across a wide range of frequencies to about 6000 Hz.

Table 7-1.   Width of Critical Band Versus Frequency

Frequency, Hz	Critical band, Hz
125	70.8
250	50.0
500	50.0
750	56.2
1000	64.0
1500	79.4
2000	100.0
3000	158.0
4000	200.0
6000	376.0
8000	501.0

Note. From "Masking of pure tones and of speech by white noise" by J. Hawkins and S. Stevens, 1950, *J. Acous. Soc. Am., 22,* pp. 6–13. Copyright 1950 by Journal of the Acoustical Society of America. Reprinted by permission.

Narrow band noise is bandpass filtered broad band noise that is defined by its center frequency, its bandwidth 3 dB down from the maximum amplitude, and the rejection rate of frequencies away from the center frequency. Examples of broad band and narrow band noise spectra are shown in Figure 7–2.

NBN is a *more efficient* masker than BBN because most of its acoustic energy is located in the region of the critical band, whereas the energy in BBN is distributed across frequencies other than those in the critical band. For this reason, NBN is also a *more effective* masker because its spectrum level is higher for any given SPL. This can be demonstrated using the noises shown in Figure 7–2, where the BBN has a bandwidth of 6000 and the NBN 200 Hz. For purposes of this demonstration we will use an overall SPL of 60 dB:

BBN	NBN
dB No = 60 − 10 log 6000	dB No = 60 − 10 log 200
log 6000 = 3.78	log 200 = 2.3
dB No = 60 − 10 (3.78)	dB No = 60 − 10 (2.3)
dB No = 60 − 37.8	dB No = 60 − 23
dB No = 22.2	dB No = 37

Because the spectrum level of the NBN is nearly 15 dB higher than that of the BBN, we would expect 15 dB more masking with the narrow band noise. That shows that it is a more effective masker. To put it another way, 14.8 dB more BBN would be necessary to pro-

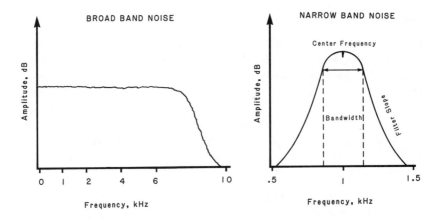

Figure 7-2. Broad band noise and narrow band noise spectra. The center frequency of the narrow band of noise is at 1000 Hz. Bandwidth and filter slope are labelled.

duce the same effective masking as the NBN (74.8 − 37.8 = 37). This indicates that the NBN is more efficient as well. If the bandwidth of a narrow band noise is less than the critical band of its center frequency, however, masking effectiveness will not be optimum.

In addition to being more efficient, the use of NBN has two important advantages. First, high masker levels may generate considerable loudness discomfort in the listener and may even lead to some temporary threshold shift. Second, at noise levels over 60 dB SPL the masker may exceed interaural attenuation levels for air conducted stimuli and, once perceptible, cause threshold shifts in the test ear. Therefore, narrow band noise is generally preferred for pure tone threshold audiometry and for other tests that use pure tones as stimuli.

HOW MUCH MASKING TO USE

Once it is apparent that masking is necessary, and a type of noise has been selected, the very important question of how much masking to use arises. This issue is by no means independent of the first two: the amount of masking necessary is determined by the amount of cross-hearing possible under some test conditions as well as by the type of masking noise used. Two methods are commonly used to determine adequate masking levels: the plateau method developed by Hood (1960) and the formula or equation method.

The Plateau Method

Consider the following situation: a subject's air conduction threshold for a pure tone is 60 dB HL on the right ear and 10 dB on the left ear. Masking is necessary to determine whether the response at 60 dB is truly that of the right ear or whether it represents cross-hearing from the left ear. Narrow band noise is introduced into the left ear at a level of 30 dB, after which the test tone is presented again at 60 dB. The subject's response—or lack of it—under the new test condition is made meaningful by reviewing some basic principles:

1. Cross-hearing occurs 40 to 60 dB above the sensorineural level of the nontest ear (NTE).
2. Masking raises threshold when both tone and masker are present in the same ear.
3. Therefore, a masker level of 30 dB is insufficient to cause cross-hearing or to raise the threshold of the test ear (TE).

What can we deduce if the subject fails to respond to the signal while the noise is present in the nontest ear? The answer lies in Principle 2: the threshold of the nontest ear has been raised so that it is no longer able to respond to the sound presented to the test ear. That is, the original response in quiet represented cross-hearing, not the threshold of the test ear. If the intensity of the tone is increased it will once again be audible. Successive increments in masking level will produce successive increments in threshold so long as the nontest ear alone is responding to the signal. In that case, *undermasking* has occurred; that is, the masking level has not raised the threshold of the nontest ear sufficiently to prevent its response to the test tone. In Figure 7–3a, auditory detection threshold has been plotted as a function of masker intensity; undermasking is indicated by thresholds that vary directly with masker level, as shown by the filled circles.

Now consider Figure 7–3b. Here, you will see that an area of undermasking has occurred at low masker levels, but that a point is reached at which threshold is unaffected by continued increases in masker intensity, again represented by the filled circles. This is the *masking plateau*. The plateau demonstrates that the signal has been heard in the test ear; the nontest ear has been successfully excluded from the listening task. Because the masking noise is present only in the nontest ear, the threshold of the test ear is unchanged.

Suppose we continue to increase the masker level? Figure 7–3c shows that the plateau does not continue indefinitely; rather, the

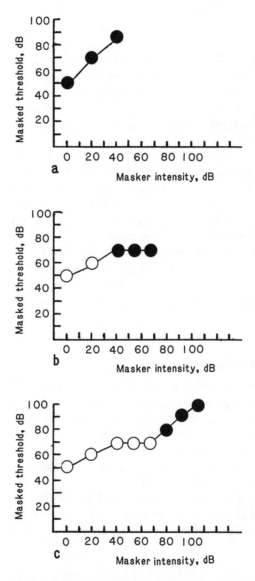

Figure 7–3. (a) Undermasking is represented when thresholds in the test ear vary directly with masker level in the nontest ear; this linear relationship demonstrates that masker and signal are present in the same ear. (b) The plateau of the function occurs when threshold is stable in spite of continued increments in masker level in the nontest ear. This shows that masker and signal are being perceived in different ears. (c) Overmasking occurs when the masker level is high enough to cross the skull by bone conduction and interfere with the tone in the test ear. Because tone and masker are once again present in the same ear, thresholds once again vary linearly with masker level.

same 1:1 relationship of masker and threshold typical of under-masking resumes. At this point, *overmasking* has started, shown by the filled circles. The masking intensity in the nontest ear over-comes interaural attenuation and therefore is present in both ears. Once the "crossed-over" masking exceeds the threshold of the test ear, its effect on detection of the test tone is the same as in the nontest ear. Each increment in masker intensity raises tone thresh-old by the same amount.

The great appeal of the plateau method of determining how much masking to use is that it is based on direct observation of the effects of masking levels on a particular subject's thresholds, rather than on a series of assumptions and models that indicate the level of masking that *should* be necessary. The plateau method also dem-onstrates very clearly when thresholds are likely to have been influ-enced by under- or overmasking and thus when their reliability should be questioned. In clinical practice, therefore, masked thresh-olds should be determined using a plateau method; the adequacy of the masking can then be cross-checked with the following post-hoc equation.

The Equation Method

There are almost as many "masking equations" as there are text-books in audiology or audiometry—perhaps more! No matter how the equations are arranged, however, all have in common terms representing the signal intensity, the amount of interaural attenua-tion, and the sensorineural level (i.e., the bone conduction sensitiv-ity) of the nontest ear. These factors, added together, define what I will call the *undesired signal* (US).

As its name implies, the undesired signal describes the level of a signal present in the test or nontest ear that interferes with accu-rate threshold measurement. It is estimated in the following way:

$$US = SI - IA - BC_{nt}$$

A test tone of 75 dB (SI) is presented to one ear. Because it is deliv-ered through an earphone it is subject to the minimum assumed interaural attenuation (IA) for air conducted signals of 40 dB. The tone then is present in the nontest ear at an intensity of about 35 dB. However, to cause any problem the level of the tone must exceed the bone conduction sensitivity of the nontest ear (BC_{nt})—that is, it must be audible. If the subject's bone conduction threshold is higher than 35 dB (in this example), the tone will not be heard; that is, cross-hearing will not occur. On the other hand, if the bone conduction threshold is lower than the level of the "crossed-over" tone, cross-hearing will occur, and masking is required. If the same signal were presented through the bone oscillator the undesired signal would be 75 dB in each ear, because IA for bone conducted signals is 0 dB.

Once the level of the US has been predicted, the minimum amount of noise required to mask it is also predictable. Because the masking noise will be delivered to the nontest ear through earphones, the air conduction threshold of the nontest ear must be considered. At this point of calculation, the minimum masking level (MML) could be expressed as follows:

$$MML = AC_{nt} + US$$

or

$$MML = AC_{nt} + (SI - IA - BC_{nt})$$

In other words, the minimum masking level must be sufficient to (1) overcome the air conduction loss of the nontest ear to be audible; and (2) prevent the NTE from responding to the undesired signal.

Finally, the minimum masking level is influenced by the type of noise used as a masker—the noise factor (NF). Because masking occurs when the total energy in a critical band exceeds the total energy in a pure tone at its center, narrow band noise can be regarded as a more effective and a more efficient masker than wide band noise. Therefore, the minimum masking level will be higher (i.e., will require more intensity) for broad band than for narrow band noise. For purposes of masking at frequencies of 1000 Hz and above, the noise factor can be calculated as 5 dB for NBN and as 15 dB for BBN (assuming the bandwidth of the NBN equals critical band for the center frequency). At frequencies below 1000 Hz, more masking is required. During the process of testing bone conduction the bone oscillator is placed on the patient's mastoid or frontal bone and the earphone used to deliver masking covers the nontest ear. When a test tone is delivered through the oscillator, its level (and, hence, the level of the undesired signal) will be correspondingly greater in the nontest ear because of the occlusion effect (OE). The occlusion effect is most prominent for low frequency stimuli; therefore, more masking is needed to be effective in that frequency range. The following examples demonstrate this principle:

Unoccluded	Occluded
US = SI – IA – BC_{nte}	US = SI + OE – IA – BC_{nte}
US = 60 – 0 – 5	US = 60 + 20 – 0 – 5
US = 55 dB	US = 75 dB

In these examples the level of the undesired signal has changed from 55 to 75 dB for a bone conducted signal of 60 dB! If the same noise factor—5 dB—were applied across frequencies without attention to the occlusion effect, the threshold of the nontest ear could not be raised sufficiently to prevent its perception of the undesired tone.

THE MASKING DILEMMA

A special problem in masking arises when a subject has bilateral conductive hearing impairment, in which bone conduction thresholds are lower than those for air conduction. The "dilemma" is that adequate masking cannot be achieved without simultaneously producing overmasking. The data presented in Figure 7–4 illustrate the problem.

Preliminary immittance testing yielded abnormal results in low static compliance and Type A_S tympanograms bilaterally in addition to a four-square acoustic reflex pattern. This combination of results suggests a bilateral conductive impairment. The air conduction thresholds are in the 60 to 65 dB HL range in each ear. Masking is necessary for air conduction because there is more than 40 dB difference between the air conduction (A/C) threshold and the projected bone conduction (B/C) sensitivity.

The masking noise must be presented at an intensity great enough to overcome the sensitivity loss in the nontest ear if it is to be audible and raise the threshold for the undesired signal in that cochlea. If the search for a masking plateau begins 10 dB above the NTE threshold, the noise would be presented initially at 70 to 75 dB. A noise of this intensity is capable of causing cross-over in the same way that a pure tone of similar intensity does. Thus, up to 30 to 35 dB of noise may be present simultaneously with the signal in the test ear. As a result, its threshold will be elevated; each increment in masking will produce an equivalent threshold elevation and a plateau will never appear. The problem is equally serious when attempting to define B/C thresholds.

The masking dilemma can be lessened by delivering the masking noise through a receiver that fits into the ear canal rather than

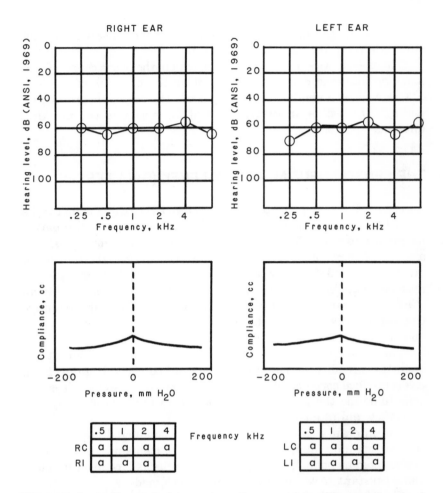

Figure 7–4. Audiometric data representing a masking dilemma. Levels of masking sufficient to overcome the attenuating effects of a middle ear disorder (indicated by the abnormal immittance results) on an air-conducted signal are, at the same time, sufficient to cause bone conduction transmission of the masker. Thus, the signal cannot be presented to the test ear independently of the masker, and threshold is raised.

through a conventional earphone. The insert receiver reduces crossover in masking in three ways: (1) sound radiation from an earphone is limited; (2) the surface area of the head in contact with the oscillating receiver is smaller than with an earphone cushion; and (3) effective masking levels can be achieved at a lower level, because the noise is delivered into a smaller cavity, thus increasing the SPL at the eardrum. If the A/C impairment in each ear is great enough, however, even the use of an insert receiver for masking will not eliminate the problem completely.

There is a way, nevertheless, in which the very cause of the masking dilemma can be used to resolve the question of cochlear (B/C) status when both ears are impaired. The *Sensorineural Acuity Level (SAL)* test is an invaluable tool for resolving the masking dilemma.

THE SENSORINEURAL ACUITY LEVEL (SAL) TEST

As Figure 7–4 demonstrated, both A/C and B/C thresholds can be shifted by masking noise that has exceeded interaural attenuation for air conduction. The extent to which air conduction thresholds are shifted depends on (1) the masking intensity; (2) the interaural attenuation; and (3) the bone conduction sensitivity of the test (non-masked) ear. As Rainville (1959) and later Jerger and Tillman (1960) demonstrated, that problem can be turned to our advantage by intentionally delivering both tone and noise to the same cochlea and observing the amount of masking that occurs.

The masking effectiveness of a noise on tones of different frequencies is readily demonstrated in normal subjects. High masking levels produce correspondingly high thresholds. Therefore, it is possible to define the normal A/C threshold in noise as a function of frequency and intensity.

The interaural attenuation for an air conducted signal varies both among individuals and as a function of frequency. If the signal is presented by bone, however, such variability is largely eliminated and a constant IA value of 0 dB can be assigned.

Therefore, if a masking noise of a set intensity were presented to a listener by bone conduction, his or her masked threshold for an air conducted tone could be predicted on the basis of the norms established for that test situation. A tested threshold that differed from the predicted threshold could then be attributed directly to middle ear abnormality, because that is the only factor that remains variable. The next series of figures will demonstrate this principle.

Figure 7–5 shows the relationship between masker intensity and masked threshold in a normal listener. Note that the masking effect does not begin until the total energy in the critical band (contained within the noise spectrum) exceeds that contained in the pure tone (*a*). After that point, masking increases linearly with increases in masker level (*b*).

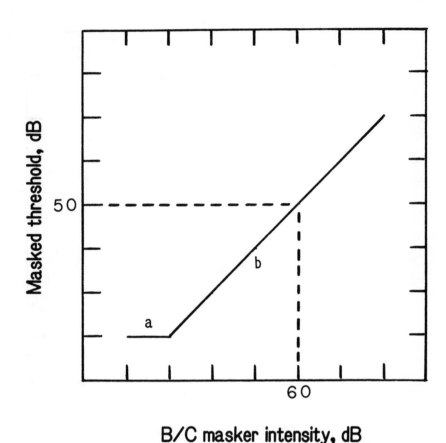

B/C masker intensity, dB

Figure 7-5. The relationship between masker intensity and masked threshold in a normal ear. Thresholds are not affected by masking until the total energy in the critical band of the noise spectrum exceeds that contained in the pure tone (a). After that point, threshold increases linearly with increases in masker level (b).

Figure 7-6 shows the effect of a conductive impairment on the masking function. Threshold is elevated because the signal is attenuated by the inefficient impedance match imposed by the middle ear disorder. Once the attenuation is overcome, however, the masking effect parallels the normal curve. This is predictable because the cochlea is functioning normally in each case and the noise is delivered by bone. The difference in dB between the masked thresholds (c) at any given point is equal to the size of the air-bone gap. Therefore, if a masked threshold of 45 dB was predicted for a cer-

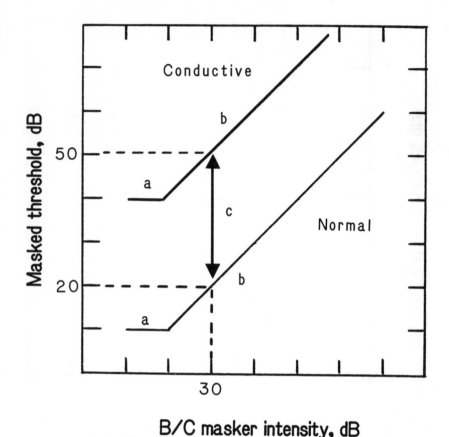

B/C masker intensity, dB

Figure 7-6. The effect of conductive hearing loss on masked threshold. Pure tone thresholds are elevated by the impedance mismatch in the middle ear. The bone conduction masking is only slightly affected by middle ear status and the masking effect is linear (b), just as it is in the normal ear.

tain masker intensity, but the measured threshold was 85 dB, an air-bone gap of 40 dB would be present.

Now consider Figure 7-7. In this example, the subject has a sensorineural impairment. Threshold for the tone is unaffected by the masker until (again) the masker energy in the critical band exceeds the energy in the signal. In this case, there is more energy in the signal than in the normal curve because it is being presented at a higher level. Thus, more masking is required. After that level has been achieved, masking proceeds on the usual 1:1 basis. When the masked thresholds of the two ears are compared, there is no difference; the air-bone gap is 0.

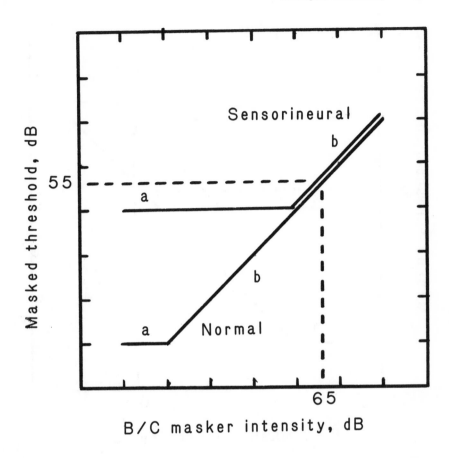

Figure 7-7. The effect of sensorineural impairment on masked threshold. Masking does not become effective until the masker energy in the critical band exceeds the energy in the signal (a). After that point, masked thresholds do not differ from the normal (b).

A third case is presented in Figure 7–8. A conductive component is manifested as a higher masked threshold than the norm, but there is a sensorineural component as well. Again, the difference between the expected and the observed masked threshold describes the size of the air-bone gap and hence, by inference, the bone conduction sensitivity.

When using the SAL technique clinically, it is necessary to bear in mind two factors. First, the contribution of the occlusion effect to bone conduction thresholds differs in conductive and sensorineural impairment. This means that the masking effectiveness will be greater in the sensorineural listener or, conversely, that the

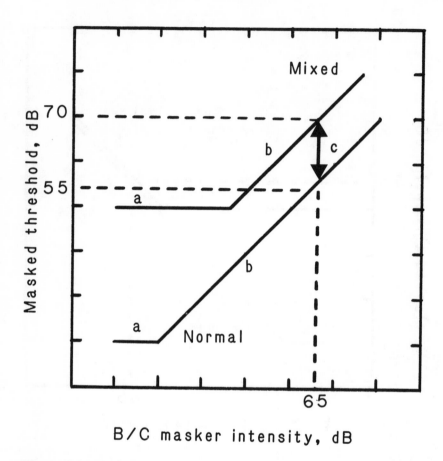

Figure 7-8. The effect of mixed hearing impairment on masked threshold. The effects of the conductive component are seen in the difference between expected and observed masked threshold (c) and the effects of the sensorineural component are seen in the higher threshold at which masking becomes effective.

cochlear reserve in the low frequencies will be underestimated in the conductive listener. This problem can be resolved either by measuring both masked and unmasked B/C thresholds or by applying a correction factor equal to the size of the normal occlusion effect at the test frequency. The second factor that may influence the accuracy of SAL measurements is that if the *unmasked* A/C threshold exceeds the normal *masked* threshold, the exact size of the conductive component cannot be determined. Thus, the SAL should be used only with patients whose A/C thresholds are lower than the SAL norm at the test frequency.

CLINICAL CONSEQUENCES OF INAPPROPRIATE MASKING

The preceding section showed that adequate masking can be demonstrated directly by establishing masked response plateaus according to the method developed by Hood (1960). The theoretical adequacy of masking can then be cross-checked by using a post-hoc equation that accounts for the status of the nontest ear, the level of the undesired signal, and the type of masking noise used. Further cross-checks on the pure tone audiogram are provided when necessary by determining the occlusion index, lateralization of a bone conducted tone (audiometric Weber), or SAL thresholds.

Using a combination of these techniques invariably lengthens testing time; for this reason some clinicians take shortcuts, such as delivering masking at a single intensity at each frequency. There are three possible outcomes to this practice: (1) results could be accurate; (2) undermasking could occur, leading to inadequate isolation of the test ear and a subsequent overestimation of its cochlear reserve; or (3) overmasking could occur, leading to interference in the test ear by crossed-over masking and a subsequent underestimation of its cochlear reserve.

Accurate and adequate masking is always very important in hearing assessment, but it becomes crucial when the patient is being evaluated for surgical treatment of a middle ear disorder. Audiometric data are used by the surgeon to help decide whether surgery is indicated; how much hearing improvement might be expected; and, in some cases, which ear should be operated on. The preoperative assessment also serves as a baseline against which postoperative results are compared.

If the main goal of masking is to isolate the test ear from the nontest ear, both undermasking and overmasking represent a failure to achieve that goal. In the case of undermasking, the test signal can be perceived by the nontest ear; overmasking interferes with perception of the signal in the test ear. Both of these situations lead to inaccurate threshold estimations.

The classic example of inappropriate masking is the "shadow curve" produced in an anacusic ("dead") ear. Panel A of Figure 7-9 shows the unmasked thresholds of such a subject. Sensitivity is within normal limits on the right ear; the left ear shows air conduction thresholds of 50 to 60 dB; and the bone conduction thresholds, although nonspecific, are in agreement with the A/C sensitivity on the right. If masking were not applied in this case, there would appear to be a moderate conductive impairment on the left ear. As

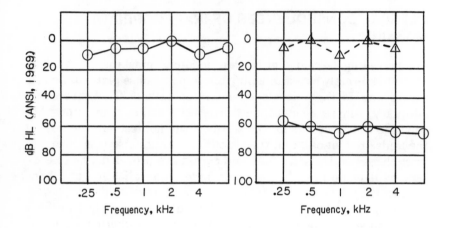

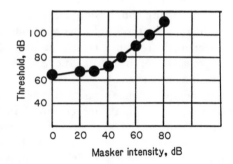

Figure 7–9. Unmasked air conduction and bone conduction thresholds of a patient with anacusis on the left ear. Note that without masking the impairment appears to be conductive; in reality, the air and bone conduction "thresholds" of the left represent the crosshearing thresholds on the right.

it happened, however, the responses observed when the signal was presented through the left earphone merely represent the bone conduction sensitivity on the right, plus the interaural attenuation at each frequency. That is, the 60 dB HL tone presented at 1000 Hz to the left ear was sufficient to cause cross-hearing on the right. The apparent "air-bone gap" is an indicant of the amount of interaural attenuation produced by that subject at 1000 Hz. When adequate masking is applied to the right ear, its threshold is raised and it can no longer respond to the signal, revealing the true nature of the loss.

The opposite case is shown in Figure 7–10. In this situation, the subject has a true conductive impairment with a large air-bone gap.

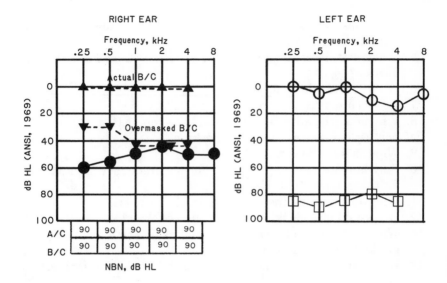

Figure 7-10. Audiometric effects of overmasking. The high levels of narrow band noise applied to the normal ear have elevated the bone conduction thresholds of the right ear, creating the impression that the loss is sensorineural rather than conductive.

Unfortunately, this condition was not identified accurately because the masking levels used were high enough to cause overmasking. The normal bone conduction thresholds were thus elevated and the impairment appeared to be sensorineural. In each of these cases, confusion could be avoided by (1) considering the results of immittance tests; (2) defining a masking plateau; and (3) using the appropriate cross-checks to verify the outcome of the bone conduction testing.

As mentioned previously, the results of pure tone audiometry are summarized on the audiogram. Chapter 8 concerns characteristics of the audiogram as a means of transmitting information efficiently and effectively.

STUDY QUESTIONS

1. How do the results of impedance audiometry allow us to make certain assumptions about the nature of a pure tone hearing loss?
2. What is meant by the "undesired signal"?
3. Distinguish between cross-over and cross-hearing.

4. Does masking the nontest ear eliminate the undesired signal? Explain your answer.
5. When is it necessary to mask for air conduction? For bone conduction?
6. What is a masking dilemma?
7. How is a masking plateau recognized?
8. Why must the air conduction and bone conduction status of the nontest ear be considered in masking?
9. What is a shadow curve?
10. Why is more masking required for low frequency signals than for those above 1000 Hz?
11. What is meant by the spectrum level of a noise?
12. How could overmasking lead to clinical error?
13. Why is narrow band noise a more efficient and a more effective masker than broad band noise?
14. How does a SAL test help overcome the masking dilemma?

Chapter 8

The Audiogram

Graphic artists know that a graph or symbol system can be the most effective means of demonstrating relationships among several factors. The audiogram is used to (1) illustrate patterns of hearing sensitivity for tones as a function of frequency; (2) compare air and bone conduction sensitivity; (3) show how a patient's hearing relates to a normative standard; (4) demonstrate interaural symmetry or asymmetry; and (5) present the results of other, related pure tone tests. The variety and complexity of this information demands the simplest graphics to avoid confusion and possible misinterpretation.

Examine Figure 8–1. Here, the data from a patient with a bilateral, asymmetrical, mixed hearing impairment are presented using the symbol system recommended by the American Speech-Language-Hearing Association (1974) and used in most clinical audiology settings. Note on the key that there are 4 symbols for air conduction and 7 for bone conduction: a total of 11! This audiogram does not transmit information effectively because it contains too many different symbols (which require the unsophisticated reader to refer to the key constantly) in a small area. Moreover, the status of each ear individually cannot be discerned without careful study.

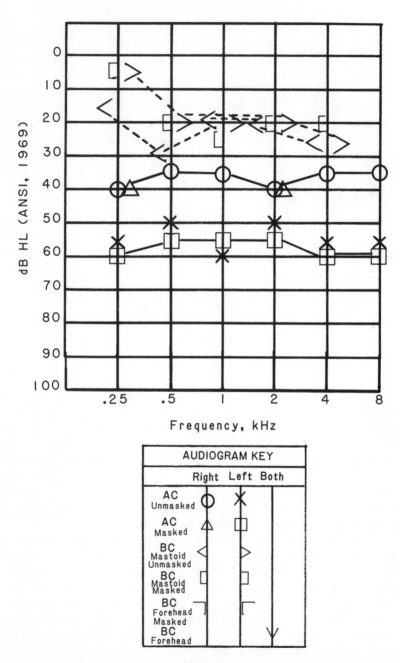

Figure 8–1. Audiometric data of a patient with a bilateral, asymmetrical mixed hearing impairment. Data are plotted using the symbol system recommended by the American Speech, Language, and Hearing Association (1974).

In Figure 8-2 the same data are presented using an audiometric symbol system proposed and used by Jerger (1976). The use of two grids, one for each ear, eliminates the need for different symbols and has an accepted precedent in the practice of plotting tympanograms on separate grids. Masking is indicated by shading in the symbol for air conduction (○) or bone conduction (△). SAL results are shown by a diamond (◊) and acoustic reflexes by a square, open for ipsilateral (□) and crossed for contralateral (⊠). In this case, there are four basic symbols. There is no question as to which bone conduction symbol belongs to which ear; in addition, the size of the air-bone gap, audiometric configuration, and interaural symmetry can be assessed at a glance. Color coding is unnecessary. The levels of masking used for air conduction and bone conduction are read with no difficulty. This audiogram transmits information in a simple, effective, and uncluttered way. The only apparent rationale for choosing the first system (it seems to me) is a stubborn clinging to tradition. The method proposed by Jerger is to be highly recommended and is used consistently throughout this book.

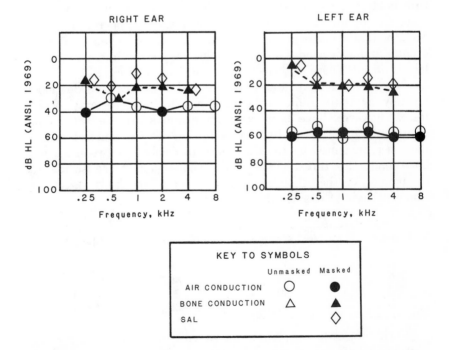

Figure 8-2. Audiometric data of the same patient in Figure 8-1 are plotted using the symbol system devised and recommended by Jerger (1976).

CLASSIFICATION OF AUDIOGRAMS

Once pure tone audiometry has been completed, the resulting audiogram can be described along three dimensions: the type of hearing impairment indicated; the severity of any impairment present; and the configuration of the hearing impairment across the audiometric range of frequencies. Classification of type is based on the air-bone gap and the B/C thresholds; classification of severity and configuration is referenced to A/C thresholds, because they are more directly related to the way in which hearing is used for purposes of speech communication.

Classification of Type

Hearing impairment is traditionally described as being conductive, sensorineural, or mixed. This classification is made by comparing air and bone conduction thresholds. If there is an air-bone gap of 10 dB or greater and bone conduction thresholds are within normal limits, the loss is described as *conductive*. If air and bone conduction thresholds are comparable (either by inference from immittance results or by direct measurement) and hearing is poorer than normal, the loss is *sensorineural*. If there is an air-bone gap of 10 dB or greater and bone conduction thresholds are poorer than normal, the loss is *mixed*. These criteria are summarized in Table 8–1.

"Pure" conductive and sensorineural losses can be described entirely by their audiometric configuration and severity. Mixed losses, however, have both conductive and sensorineural components and thus require further definition. The conductive component is represented by the difference in decibels between air and bone conduction thresholds, or the air-bone gap. The sensorineural component, on the other hand, is represented by the bone conduction sensitivity. Consider the following cases:

Subject	A/C average	B/C average	Classification
A	50	5	Conductive
B	50	45	Sensorineural
C	50	20	Mixed
D	50	35	Mixed

Each subject has the same sensitivity impairment by air conduction but different degrees of impairment for bone-conducted signals. Subject A's hearing loss is purely conductive, which means

Table 8-1.   Classification of Hearing Impairment

Type	Air-Bone Gap	B/C Thresholds
Conductive	> 10 dB	< 15 dB
Sensorineural	≤ 10 dB	≥ 15 dB
Mixed	> 10 dB	> 15 dB

that the entire impairment can be accounted for by inefficient impedance matching in the middle or outer ear. Subject B's impairment is purely sensorineural and can be accounted for by abnormal structure or function of the cochlea or auditory nerve. Subject C has a mixed loss: the conductive component is 30 dB (air-bone gap = 50 − 20 = 30 dB), whereas the sensorineural component, represented by the bone conduction thresholds, is 20 dB. In this case, most of the hearing impairment can be accounted for by middle ear dysfunction and relatively little by the cochlea or auditory nerve. The opposite conclusion can be drawn from the data of Subject D, who also has a mixed loss: the conductive component is only 15 dB (50–35), whereas the sensorineural component is 35 dB. If each of these two subjects were treated successfully for their middle ear disorders, Subject C would enjoy greater improvement of hearing than would Subject D, whose thresholds cannot be substantially improved beyond his 35 dB sensorineural level. This information can be valuable to otologic surgeons as they consider the risk-benefit ratio in planning surgical correction of middle ear abnormalities that are not life-threatening.

Classification of Severity

Hearing impairment is classified as mild, moderate, severe, and profound. Classification can be made on the basis of sensitivity at a single frequency of interest or on the basis of average sensitivity across several frequencies—the "pure tone average" or PTA. The average of air conduction thresholds at 500, 1000, and 2000 Hz is designated PTA_1; thresholds averaged across 1000, 2000, and 4000 Hz are designated PTA_2. Table 8-2 summarizes the ranges of thresholds included in each category of severity.

These classifications, like most other kinds of "pigeonholing," can lead to some serious misunderstandings about a patient's hearing impairment. One common mistake is to equate the name of the category (e.g., "normal," "mild") with the seriousness of the audi-

Table 8-2. Classification of Severity of Hearing Loss

dB HL	Classification
0–10	Normal
15–40	Mild
45–65	Moderate
70–90	Severe
>90	Profound

tory disorder. Any person who has experienced a 35 to 40 dB hearing loss will tell you there is nothing "mild" about it when listening conditions are poor; conversely, very serious auditory disorders are often present as a result of brain stem or auditory cortex pathology, despite the patient's having quite normal pure tone sensitivity. A second error, often made by patients, is to equate threshold level with "percentage of hearing loss." Thus, a 60 dB loss would be called "60 percent hearing loss." This concept has arisen from the attempts of various compensation boards to reduce the concept of auditory handicap to a single number for purposes of awarding compensation. Its validity is limited by the fact that the impact of a given degree of hearing impairment on an individual varies greatly according to many factors, such as listening situation, lipreading ability, occupational needs for hearing, lifestyle, etiologic factors, and accompanying symptoms of the disorder. For example, two patients may have identical audiograms, showing a 30 to 35 dB high frequency sensorineural impairment. Both would be classified as having 12 percent impairment. However, if one man made his living tuning pianos whereas the other worked as a farmer, the impact of the loss would be quite different for the two men. Moreover, the concept of losing a given "percentage" of hearing is tied to the norms for audiometric zero rather than to any innate capacity for hearing.

Classification of Audiogram Configuration

Once the type and degree of hearing impairment is known, a study of the pattern of sensitivity loss across several frequencies—the audiogram configuration—can provide supplementary information about the underlying nature of the disorder. Most audiogram configurations fall into three basic categories: flat; rising; and sloping. Examples of these configurations are presented in Figure 8-3.

The flat audiogram shows variation in thresholds of less than 15 dB across the range of frequencies tested. For example, an audio-

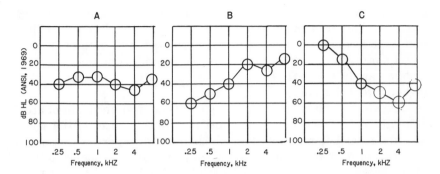

Figure 8-3. Common audiogram configurations. A: Flat configuration. B: Rising configuration. C: Sloping configuration.

gram in which all thresholds from 250 to 8000 Hz fall within the range of 35 to 50 dB HL would be described as flat.

The rising configuration is characterized by greater hearing impairment for the low frequency tones than for high frequencies. This is a relatively uncommon type of configuration and can appear on both a conductive and a sensorineural basis.

The audiogram with a sloping configuration shows better sensitivity in the low frequencies than in the high frequencies. A configuration is said to be "steeply" or "precipitously" sloping if the thresholds at adjacent frequencies differ by >20 dB/octave. The sloping configuration is quite common and is typical of many types of sensorineural disorders, although certain middle ear disorders may produce this pattern as well.

These configurations can be accounted for by recalling some principles of physiological acoustics. Consider, for example, the sloping configuration, in which sensitivity for high frequency stimuli is impaired. If the impairment is found to be conductive, a sloping configuration suggests an impedance mismatch related to increased mass reactance in the middle or outer ears, and therefore may be described as a *mass tilt*. When the reactance due to stiffness is lower than that due to mass, acoustic impedance varies directly with the frequency of the signal. That is, systems characterized by high mass reactance transmit high frequencies inefficiently. The sloping conductive hearing impairment can be produced by either relative or absolute increases in mass. In the case of an ossicular discontinuity, the mass of the ossicles remains unchanged from the normal state but stiffness is greatly reduced by the disruption of the ossicular joint. Thus, the relative contributions of mass and stiffness to the total impedance are abnormal. An absolute increase in mass, however, would be produced by a middle ear tumor (e.g., a cholesteatoma) or a thickened tympanic membrane. In each condition, high frequency stimuli must be presented with greater intensity to overcome the transmission inefficiency imposed by the middle ear disorder. Higher stimulus intensities are recorded as higher thresholds on the audiogram.

The underlying bases of a sloping sensorineural impairment are quite different. In this case, we must look to the status of the sensory and neural elements of the cochlea and eighth nerve to account for elevated pure tone thresholds. Recall that high frequency stimuli are received most efficiently by the hair cells located toward the base of the cochlea. If those cells are damaged or missing, the sound intensity must be raised to increase the amplitude of the traveling wave on the basilar membrane and thus stimulate other receptor cells. Again, these high signal intensities necessary to achieve audibility are recorded as higher thresholds.

A conductive impairment having a rising configuration suggests that there is increased stiffness in the middle ear, such as that found with ossicular fixation. Remember that the influence of the stiffness reactance component of total acoustic impedance varies inversely with the frequency of the sound. That is, low frequency sounds are transmitted less efficiently than high frequency sounds through a system dominated by stiffness. Sometimes this audiometric configuration is referred to as having a *stiffness tilt*. A rising sensorineural impairment is often associated with Meniere's disease, a condition also known to alter stiffness on the basis of increased fluid pressure in the cochlear partition.

Audiogram configuration should never be regarded as "proof" of certain types of pathology. There are many sources of variance and error in hearing assessment procedures that can alter the appearance and subsequent interpretation of audiograms. Some of these sources are discussed in the next chapter.

STUDY QUESTIONS

1. What arguments could you present to your employer in support of changing the audiograms used in your clinic to the simplified form presented in this chapter?

2. Why is the concept of "percentage of hearing loss" likely to be confusing and inaccurate?

3. Why would a patient with ossicular discontinuity have a high frequency conductive hearing impairment?

Chapter 9

Sources of Variance in Pure Tone Audiometry

As we have established, pure tone audiometry in a clinical setting measures a subject's relative rather than absolute auditory thresholds. The thresholds obtained in this way represent the subject's auditory sensitivity as influenced both by his or her physiological status and by a number of other factors present at the time of the test; thus they have an inherent variance. Some of these factors can lead to error in threshold measurement and thus to incorrect conclusions about the subject's auditory status. The sources of error in pure tone audiometry are discussed in this chapter. Other factors are responsible for variance in test behavior for a given subject within or between any given test session(s). Some sources of variance in audiometric testing are shown in Table 9–1.

These factors, interacting, largely determine how closely a subject's relative thresholds approximate his or her "true" or absolute thresholds at any given testing session. Some of them, if unrecognized, lead to error. Consider, for example, equipment calibration. At most frequencies audiometer output is permitted to fall within ± 3 dB of the ANSI standard for that frequency. Thus, if the standard for 1 kHz is 7 dB SPL, the actual output can range between 4 and 10 dB SPL for audiometric 0. This would create a variance of

Table 9-1.   Sources of Variance in Audiometric Testing

Room	Noise levels Temperature Reverberation Calibration	
Equipment	Calibration: Stimulus:	Frequency Intensity Reference standard Rise-fall times Duration
	Distortion Voltage stability Intermittent faults Earphone:	 Circumaural Supra-aural Hard Soft Insert Frequency response Maximum output
Tester	Attention Response criteria Motivation Personality:	 Interpretation Expectancy bias
Test technique	Ascending, descending, hybrid Stimulus duration Manual or semi-automatic Response-indicating method Instructions Interstimulus intervals	
Earphone-subject interactions	Comfort Leak from phones Standing waves in canal Collapsing canals	
Subject	Motivation Comprehension of instructions Judgmental criteria Detection variance Learning effect Personality Circadian effects Attention Comfort Fatigue Colds Cerumen Temporary threshold shift True fluctuating hearing impairment	
Tester-subject interactions		

From Stephens, 1981.

about 5 dB, an acceptable deviation. If, however, the output at the same frequency were 20 dB SPL when the attenuator is set at 0, a 10 dB error would be made by using the dial reading to indicate threshold. Moreover, output reference standards vary slightly, depending on the type of earphone used to deliver the signal; calibration of an audiometer that uses TDH-39 earphones to a TDH-49 standard is an obvious error, although not a serious one. Patients who are in great physical discomfort from illness or drugs usually are less interested than the audiologist in the accuracy and reliability of their responses.

There is probably no greater source of variance in the entire battery of tests than in bone conduction measurement. For this reason alone, the use of immittance audiometry as the routine first step of the assessment is recommended. As shown previously, a completely normal set of immittance results rules out the contribution of a middle ear disorder to the total auditory impairment and thus obviates the need for bone conduction testing. An exception to this principle should be made if collapsing ear canals are suspected. In this case, an air-bone gap would appear, because the ear canals would be collapsed by the presence of the earphones but not by the bone oscillator. The necessary confirming evidence of a conductive disorder would be absent from the immittance results, however, unless a horizontal pattern of acoustic reflex abnormality appeared.

Bone conduction thresholds are influenced by many external factors: type of oscillator; surface area of the oscillator; position on the mastoid process or on the frontal bone (forehead); and pressure of the oscillator against the skull. Of these, the most common source of clinical variance is in the placement of the oscillator.

There is no doubt that frontal placement of the oscillator offers a more stable position, has less variability in the tissue density underlying the oscillator, and has greater test-retest reliability than mastoid placement (Goodhill, Dirks, and Malmquist, 1970; Studebaker, 1962). There is also a significant advantage to frontal placement in that it prevents the clinician from making the erroneous assumption that a bone oscillator placed on the right mastoid, for example, is actually testing the right ear. Nevertheless, most audiologists continue to place the bone oscillator on the mastoid process. When this is done, thresholds may be underestimated if the oscillator contacts the pinna and thus transmits vibrotactile information as a cue. Similarly, placement of the oscillator too high or too low (front or back) on the mastoid may change thresholds as much as 15 dB. Patients with very oily skin may experience slippage of the oscillator during the test, with resulting fluctuation or variability in thresholds. Headbands that are too loose or large for a patient's head exert force against the head that is insufficient to oscillate the skull effectively at all frequencies; again, the result will be inaccurate threshold estimates.

Another, less frequently discussed source of potential error in bone conduction testing lies in an oscillator that has been damaged by dropping or being hit, but which may be calibrated only infrequently with an artificial mastoid. Regular biological calibration of the bone oscillator should alert the clinician to the possibility of equipment error.

Patients should receive special instructions for responding to bone-conducted signals. Some patients are confused by lateralization effects caused by conductive or sensorineural impairment and defer a response until their perception seems "right." For example, a patient with an asymmetrical sensorineural hearing impairment will lateralize an unmasked bone conduction signal to his or her better ear. If the bone oscillator is on the opposite ear, the patient may not respond until the sound is perceived in that ear. Conversely, conductive impairment causes a bone-conducted sound to lateralize toward the ear with the greatest air-bone gap; in this case, the patient may again become confused by the seeming discrepancy between the ear receiving the signal and the ear perceiving the sound.

In the assessment of conductive hearing impairment, bone conduction measurements are irreplaceable; in other circumstances, bone conduction can be realistically viewed as the weakest link in the chain of audiometric tests. For this reason, the cross-checks to bone conduction threshold information—the audiometric Weber test, the occlusion index, and the SAL—assume even greater importance in interpreting the clinical data. Finally, one seldom-discussed source of variance exists in the size of the external ear canal. The output of audiometers is calibrated with the earphone applied to a 6 cm^3 coupler, a volume representing the average space enclosed between the speaker of a supra-aural earphone and the tympanic membrane. Many subjects, however, have canal volumes that are larger or smaller than 6 cm^3. As you will recall, sound pressure level varies inversely with cavity size. This means that SPL at the tympanic membrane is greater in a smaller canal than in a larger canal, even though the earphone output was identical. The difference is more important at some frequencies than others, because a second effect of changing ear canal volume and length is a change in its resonant frequency: a smaller volume resonates at a higher frequency than a larger volume.

SOURCES OF ERROR

The accuracy of pure tone audiometry rests on the skill of the examiner, the cooperation of the subject, and meticulous maintenance of the test equipment and environment to meet ANSI standards. Shortcomings in these areas introduce error to the test results. The presence of error is often signaled by inconsistencies in test results: between observed communication ability and pure tone sensitivity; between the results of immittance and pure tone audiometry; between one trial and another within the test sequence; between observed and expected test behavior. Dr. Charles Berlin, a wise teacher and clinician, advises the examiner to "suspect yourself first, your equipment next, and the subject last" in trying to unravel inconsistent test behavior. That is, unusual or inconsistent test results are more likely to arise from examiner or equipment error than from some exotic condition or motivation in the patient. Berlin's succinct advice leads us to consider more closely the sources of error in the clinician, the test equipment and environment, and the subject.

Clinician Sources of Error

Unless a subject is an experienced "test-taker" or is feigning some auditory status, he or she will usually do exactly as the clinician instructs. If the instructions have been vague, the subject's behavior is likely to be maddeningly vague as well, because he or she was not given enough structure for a firm response criterion. The clinician must state, in a clear and understandable way, exactly what the subject is expected to do in response to a tone: when to respond, how to respond, how long and how often to respond, and so forth. Under ordinary circumstances the subject should also be told what to expect during the test so that he or she will not spend time wondering why the tone is present only in one ear or why the pitch of the tone has changed, rather than attending to the task. If a severe hearing impairment is obvious, special care must be taken in ensuring that the subject understands the instructions.

After the instructions have been given and understood, the clinician fits the headset. Herein lies another potential source of error: if the headset is too loose or too small, the earphone speaker will not be in line with the external auditory meatus; earphones can be placed on the wrong ears or in such a way as to collapse the ear canal. In each of these situations some serious errors in test results can be expected.

When the earphones are properly seated, the clinician returns to the audiometer to begin the test. A few seconds spent looking at the various control settings, hands in lap, can eliminate other sources of error. Check to see that the signal parameters (i.e., frequency, intensity, pulsed or continuous) are correct. Make certain the correct output has been chosen—earphone, bone oscillator, loudspeaker, right or left. If masking is desired, the channel through which it will be directed should be on, and its output level and destination chosen. These few seconds spent asking "Can I do what I intend to do?" will save even the most experienced examiner time and trouble.

Once the test is under way, the clinician must guard against giving visual or timing cues to the patient. A steady pattern of tone presentations, such as one every 1 to 2 seconds, encourages the subject to pick up the same pattern, with the result that it becomes difficult to sort out the true and false positive responses. Of course, a tone presentation followed by a questioning look at the subject will lead to the same situation.

Finally, there are clinician errors that can only be described as negligent. These include beginning the test without applying the earphones or bone oscillator, failing to turn on the equipment power, testing the same ear twice, failing to turn on the masking channel, leaving the door to the test room ajar, and similar errors. Most clinicians will admit to one or more of these sorts of errors during their careers.

Consider the following anecdote. A student clinician was beginning one of his first audiometric assessments with a "real patient" rather than a fellow student. He instructed her in meticulous detail and began the test after a careful survey of the audiometer control settings. The patient did not begin to respond on the right ear until the signal was 80 dB HL or higher at each frequency. The same results were obtained for the left ear. The student was puzzled: "I didn't think her hearing was that bad when I was taking her history." At last he saw the problem: the earphones were still hanging securely on the wall bracket, rather than being on the patient's head. With extraordinary poise, he strolled back into the test chamber, beamed at the patient and said, "That was very good. Now we'll do the same thing with these earphones." The moral of this true story is that in most instances, patients are unaware that errors have been made by the examiner. Although it is crucial for the examiner to recognize and then correct such errors, it is equally important to maintain composure and control of the test situation so that the patient's confidence in the examiner will remain unshaken.

Equipment and Environmental Sources of Error

The greatest single source of error in audiometric assessment probably arises from improperly calibrated equipment. Regular output calibration checks must be routine to give meaning to the otherwise arbitrary numbers on the attenuator dials. In addition, listening checks of all equipment should be planned for the start of each clinical day. Such checks are designed to identify problems in attenuator linearity, signal distortion, "cross-talk" (a signal present in both earphones when only one is activated), audible clicks, static or 60 Hz hum, and so forth. Equipment problems such as frayed earphone cables can also be identified.

The effects of some equipment problems are not inconsequential. For example, a nonlinear attenuator will prevent accurate threshold measurement. Thomas and colleagues (1969) wrote of their discovery of an audiometer that did not attenuate below 50 dB; this meant that any person with hearing between – 10 and 50 dB HL would seem to have thresholds of – 10 dB! Similarly, an audiometer with no output below a dial reading of 25 dB would never demonstrate normal hearing. When frequency distortion occurs, the "pure" tone may be transformed into a broad spectrum sound lacking frequency specificity. A high frequency hearing impairment, therefore, would go undetected as the subject responded to the low frequency components of the distorted tone. Frayed or partially interrupted earphone cords often result in an intermittent signal; thus, the patient may not respond consistently to test stimuli. This can lead to a false impression of nonorganic hearing impairment or elevated thresholds.

The test environment is equally important. A test room equipped with a noisy exhaust fan or one located next to an elevator shaft may be noisy enough to produce masking of low frequencies. A room that is inadequately ventilated, on the other hand, may be very quiet and very warm—conditions that encourage dozing or produce discomfort, both of which are effective distractors from the task of trying to detect tones at threshold.

Patient Sources of Error

Auditory sensitivity is measured by two general methods. In one, a signal is presented and an involuntary, automatic response is recorded. This type of procedure is often referred to as an *objective or physiological* test. An example of this method might be recording the compound action potential from the auditory nerve. The threshold at which a response can be elicited is determined by the signal characteristics and by the physiological state of the auditory system up to that level. The second method, sometimes called *subjective or behavioral,* requires the subject to make a voluntary response when a signal is presented. In this case, threshold depends on an additional factor: the decision of the subject to respond. The signal intensity at which that decision is made depends on the response criterion adopted by the subject and can be influenced by a number of external and internal factors. The instruction, "Raise your hand [or push the button] as soon as you hear the sound" could be interpreted in the following ways:

1. Raise your hand as soon as you detect anything different from silence.

2. Raise your hand as soon as you think you hear a tone.

3. Raise your hand as soon as you're sure a tone is present.

4. Raise your hand as soon as a tone of some loudness is heard.

Each of these interpretations reflects a different response criterion and will result in a different "threshold" being recorded. Therefore, the criterion, whether generated by the examiner or by the subject, represents a source of error in threshold measurement. That is, the points on an audiogram intended to represent detection thresholds may actually represent identification or even most comfortable loudness thresholds. Even when very precise instructions are given by the examiner, criterion differences can be expected. Elderly and very young subjects often adopt a more strict response criterion (i.e., waiting to respond until certain that the signal is present). When a patient is afflicted with tinnitus in the test ear, his or her responses may become erratic or inconsistent as the test frequency approaches that of the tinnitus. The rate of false positive responses may increase and thresholds appear to return abruptly to the normal range. The problem may be resolved or lessened by using a pulsed rather than continuous tone; by asking the patient to report the number of pulses heard during a given interval; or by asking the patient to report when he or she begins to experience confusion between the tinnitus and the test signal.

   A less frequently encountered source of error is the presence of retrocochlear eighth nerve disorder, often characterized by abnormal adaptation ("tone decay"). Very rapid adaptation during the presentation of a continuous tone (and a subsequent recovery period) produces spurious threshold elevation. In this case, as with tinnitus, changing to a pulsed tone presentation may help to establish thresholds because the pulsed tones are usually too brief to be affected by adaptation. Although accurate definition of thresholds is very important for the interpretation of other test results, it is equally important for the examiner to be aware that adaptation is present. This can be achieved by instructing the patient to respond to the signal immediately, for its entire duration, and to report any loss or change of tonality in a signal.

Impairment of pure tone sensitivity is not characteristic of central auditory disorders. As Jerger and colleagues (1969) have noted, however, temporal summation is gravely abnormal when a temporal lobe disorder is present. In that instance, pure tone thresholds may appear to be elevated when pulsed or brief continuous tones are presented.

Immittance audiometry provides a wealth of information about possible sites of auditory disorder; pure tone audiometry is used to reject certain preliminary hypotheses about auditory status and to support others by defining the type, severity, and configuration of sensitivity impairment. The next stage of the basic assessment, speech audiometry, also provides useful diagnostic information, but, perhaps more importantly, it allows us to approach the ultimate issue about auditory dysfunction: its effect on speech communication.

STUDY QUESTIONS

1. Compare the advantages and disadvantages of measuring bone conduction thresholds from the mastoid process versus from the forehead.

2. What is the difference between a "physiological" and a "behavioral" test of auditory function? Give an example of each.

3. In medical diagnosis, a common cliché is, "When you hear hoofbeats, think of horses, not zebras." How does this principle apply to auditory assessment?

4. What are some ways of overcoming the distracting or confusing influence of tinnitus during pure tone testing?

Chapter 10

Speech Audiometry

The assessment procedures described in the preceding chapters are based on the use of the simplest acoustic units—sinusoids or pure tones—as stimuli. As diagnostic tools, such tests are efficient indicants of peripheral dysfunction, but their usefulness lessens as auditory structure and function become more complex. As tools for predicting auditory handicap, designing aural (re)habilitation programs, or assessing the impact of hearing impairment on communication, pure tone tests are of limited usefulness.

Speech audiometry has the advantages of *versatility* in its applicability to diagnostic or rehabilitative purposes, *relevance* to the impact of hearing impairment on daily function, and *sensitivity* to central auditory dysfunction. The purpose of the following sections is to discuss the principles underlying the use of speech materials in clinical hearing assessment, describe some materials presently available or in use, and examine the significance of speech audiometry within the context of the test battery.

PRINCIPLES OF SPEECH AUDIOMETRY

We are all familiar with the fable of the blind men and the elephant: each man attempted to describe the massive beast entirely in terms of its tail, trunk, or leg, those being the only parts each had "tested." Like the elephant, speech understanding is a sum of many parts, which may be affected in many ways, or not at all, by hearing impairment. What, then, *is* the effect of hearing impairment on speech processing? The most accurate answer may be, "It depends."

Refer to Figure 10–1. A three-dimensional matrix is shown: one dimension represents levels or types of speech stimuli—phonemes, words, sentences, and so forth. A second dimension represents the type of auditory behavior required of the listener—detection, recognition, discrimination, and so forth. The third dimension presents various conditions under which a specified response to a given stimulus must occur. Each block in the matrix represents a different task, which could be viewed as some aspect of "speech processing." In this example, there are 288 different combinations of stimulus, response, and listening conditions (8 × 6 × 6) that vary along a continuum from basic to complex (or difficult) and require different levels of processing, some of which are nonauditory. For example, even a person with the most profound hearing impairment could detect many speech sounds by visual cues alone ("look alone"), but detection in a strictly auditory mode, as on the telephone, would be considerably poorer. Similarly, a person with normal hearing might have excellent speech understanding while talking on the telephone in a quiet office, but have trouble conducting the same conversation at a noisy party. It would be misleading to characterize a listener's ability to use speech signals on the basis of only one of these tasks, such as the phone conversation at the party or, at the other extreme, the deaf person's ability to detect speech visually. To return to the original analogy, we would be describing only the trunk or the tail of the elephant.

Conversely, it is clearly impractical to attempt to test each of the functions represented by the matrix. Even if each test took only 1 minute to administer, nearly 5 hours would be required! Therefore, a limited number of speech materials and tasks are selected to meet the specific goals of the assessment—diagnostic, habilitative, or predictive—and to address the speech communication problems of which the patient has complained.

Purposes of Speech Audiometry

Speech audiometry can be used for two purposes: (1) to contribute further diagnostic information in differentiating among various conditions; or (2) to assess speech processing for the purpose of com-

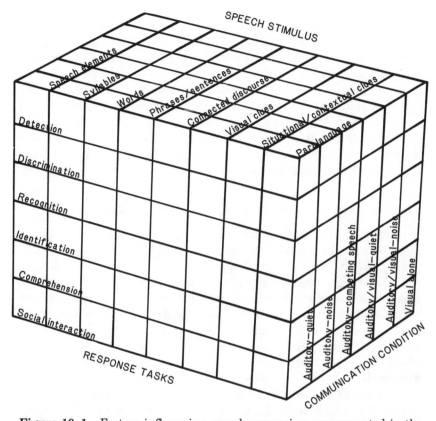

Figure 10-1. Factors influencing speech processing are presented in the form of a three-way matrix. One dimension represents types of speech stimuli; a second dimension represents the listener response behavior; the third dimension represents modality conditions in which the response to the stimulus must occur. With permission, Tobin, 1978.

munication in daily life. As Lyregaard, Robinson, and Hinchcliffe (1976) have pointed out in their monograph on speech audiometry, there is no reason to assume that a speech test suitable for one objective is suitable for the other. If speech materials are used for strictly diagnostic purposes, they need not have any relevance to daily communication or degree of handicap; their value lies in the efficiency with which they differentiate among the possible disorders. On the other hand, there is little reason to use materials that are highly sensitive to certain disorders for purposes of assessing communication efficiency if treatment and management protocols are based on degree of handicap, not on site of disorder. As an extreme example, assume that a certain disorder is characterized by the inability to identify the phoneme /s/. The optimum *diagnos-*

tic test for that disorder would consist of many trials in which the patient's ability to identify /s/ would be tested under different conditions. Such a test, however, would have little applicability in predicting the impact of the disorder on daily communication function; there are so many other sources of information available in the speech signal that the /s/ deficit would be trivial. Conversely, a test designed to assess degree of handicap would include measures of the patient's ability to use visual and contextual cues in processing speech, cues that would override subtle differences in auditory function related to specific disorders.

The Concept of Redundancy in Speech Audiometry

According to a standard dictionary, *redundancy* means an "overabundance or excessive profusion or proliferation in excess of [basic] requirements; superfluous." In literature and journalism, redundancy may detract from effective communication; in speech perception, redundancy is the factor that probably accounts for the surprisingly high resistance of speech to the distortions imposed by unfavorable listening situations or by auditory dysfunction. The pioneering work of Bocca and Calearo (1963) presented the concepts of *intrinsic and extrinsic redundancy* as they apply to speech audiometry.

In its normal state, the auditory system, like many systems of the body, is highly redundant. This means that sensory information is duplicated through rich neural interconnections at several levels between the cochlear nuclei and the auditory cortex. Such an arrangement allows auditory processing to continue in an essentially normal manner even if discrete lesions occur along the pathway. When the system is completely normal it is said to have a high degree of *intrinsic redundancy;* pathological conditions reduce that redundancy by limiting the number of duplicate channels available to transmit information. The degree to which intrinsic redundancy is reduced would depend on the site and the extent of the lesion.

If the auditory system is rich in the number of channels available to handle the same information, speech is rich in the number of cues available to specify the same information; it has a high degree of *extrinsic redundancy.* Speech remains intelligible across a wide range of speakers and listening conditions with the assistance of an abundance of acoustic, phonemic, linguistic, contextual, and suprasegmental cues. The cues are often duplicative and may assume different levels of importance in different conditions. For example, following a conversation at a noisy gathering may depend more highly on contextual and visual cues when acoustic and phonemic information is lessened by the masking effect of background noise. Extrinsic redundancy in a speech signal can be reduced in several ways; it can be filtered, played against a background of noise, time-compressed, interrupted, and presented at intensity levels close to threshold so that acoustic information is not uniformly available.

The concepts of intrinsic and extrinsic redundancy are most applicable to diagnostic speech audiometry, particularly in seeking to identify central auditory dysfunction. A system with normal intrinsic redundancy can process a signal of limited extrinsic redundancy reasonably well; most of us can understand speech in noise or filtered speech, follow the cartoon Chipmunks' time-compressed speech, and carry on softly whispered conversations in the classroom. Similarly, a signal possessing its full complement of extrinsic redundancy can be processed with little loss of information through a system having limited intrinsic redundancy. If, however, the signal has limited extrinsic redundancy, it will be processed only with extraordinary difficulty through that same limited system. Thus, the strategy in searching for evidence of central auditory dysfunction, as Bocca and Calearo (1963) demonstrated, is to present low redundancy materials "sensitized" to the presence of an impaired, poorly redundant system.

SPEECH AUDIOMETRY MEASURES

Many speech materials can be used to probe different levels of auditory function and thus can be used for several purposes. A brief description of these levels will make the ensuing discussion more meaningful.

1. *Detection* requires only a judgment as to whether a signal is minimally audible, without any further classification. It is used as a measure of auditory sensitivity.
2. *Discrimination* means making a judgment of "same" or "different" between a target stimulus and one or more comparison stimuli. It does not necessarily require correct identification or even recognition, only differentiation between or among stimuli.
3. *Recognition* involves a report of the nature of the signal or message that can be matched to a set of target messages (i.e., selecting the word presented from a list of alternatives).

4. *Identification* is essentially the same as recognition with the exception that the set of alternatives is unspecified or open-ended.
5. *Comprehension* implies a response indicating that the message has been understood, as in replying to a question or performing a requested action.

Simple stimuli such as nonsense syllables, words, and phonemes are most often used in tests of speech detection, recognition, discrimination, and identification, but they are not suitable for tests of comprehension. By contrast, the sentences and phrases most suitable for testing comprehension are usually too complex to be used for assessment of lower level functioning.

Many terms are used in the literature to describe auditory processing of speech materials; unfortunately, not all are accurate or appropriate. The following is a list of terms used to describe the same test of monosyllable identification:

- Speech intelligibility
- Speech discrimination
- Word intelligibility
- Word discrimination
- Word recognition
- PB [word] score

To avoid confusion, it is best to reserve the term *intelligibility* for describing the quality of speech *production* rather than speech *perception*. This is especially important when hearing impaired individuals are under discussion: "He has very poor speech intelligibility" has two distinct interpretations. One is that the person's speech production is poorly intelligible to other listeners; this might be expected in a situation in which severe bilateral hearing impairment has been present for a long time. The second interpretation is that the person has performed poorly on a task requiring him or her to identify monosyllable words at a suprathreshold level.

It is similarly inaccurate to describe a word identification task as "speech discrimination" or even "word discrimination" because comparison between a standard and a test stimulus is not a part of the identification task. Finally, as Figure 10-1 illustrates, there are many variables that affect the perception of speech signals. To describe the results of a single test as being representative of a listener's ability to process *speech* would be about as accurate as drawing conclusions about that person's general motor skills based on a handwriting sample. With these cautions in mind, we will now consider some specific measures of speech processing.

Threshold Measurements

Pure tone thresholds are established to determine a patient's sensitivity to simple stimuli of discrete frequencies and to serve as a foundation for describing the severity of impairment. The ultimate significance of any given hearing impairment, however, lies in the extent to which hearing of speech for communication is affected. Therefore, the auditory assessment often includes some threshold measure for speech stimuli.

The *speech detection threshold* (SDT) or *speech awareness threshold* (SAT) is the level in decibels at which a listener is aware of speech 50 percent of the time. Recognition or identification of what is being said is not necessary; only a minimal awareness of sound is required. The nature of this task is most closely related to the principle underlying pure tone threshold measurement—detection of a change from silence. Awareness thresholds are often established using connected speech, but single words or digits may be used as well. There are two reasons why awareness thresholds are not used routinely in the auditory assessment. First, the information yielded is limited to an estimate of auditory sensitivity in the 500 to 4000 Hz range. Second, a more relevant question about the impact of hearing impairment on speech communication is related to how efficiently speech can be perceived at suprathreshold, rather than threshold, levels. For these reasons, assessment time is rarely devoted to such a procedure unless the subject is unwilling or unable to participate in other types of threshold measurements.

The second type of speech threshold is often referred to as the *speech reception threshold* (SRT). Many clinicians, however, have adopted the more descriptive term *spondee threshold* (ST), which indicates the type of speech stimulus used to establish the threshold. Spondee words are two-syllable words in which equal stress is applied to each syllable: baseball, cowboy, toothbrush, and so forth. Because the two syllables are equally stressed, and because syllabic stress is conveyed (in part) by vocal intensity changes during production of a word (e.g., *pic*nic versus pic*nic*), phonemic information should be uniformly available in each syllable. The actual intensity of each word varies with the formant frequencies of its component phonemes and their relative intensities (Rupp, 1980). Spondee words have the additional feature of being highly redundant or predictable words; that is, they can be identified with a high degree of accuracy even if only part of the word is heard. A list of spondee words used in clinical assessment is presented in Table 10–1. The ST establishes the level in dB at which spondee words can be identified correctly (usually repeated aloud by the patient) 50 percent of

Table 10–1.   Spondee Word Lists

airplane	armchair
baseball	backbone
blackboard	birthdate
cowboy	cookbook
drawbridge	doormat
duck pond	earthquake
eardrum	eyebrow
horseshoe	greyhound
hot dog	hardware
ice cream	headlight
mousetrap	inkwell
northwest	mushroom
oatmeal	nutmeg
pancake	outside
playground	padlock
railroad	stairway
sunset	toothbrush
whitewash	woodwork

the time. In a sense, the spondee threshold could be regarded as a more meaningful indicant of sensitivity for speech. That is, it defines some minimal level at which information can be received through a speech signal, in contrast to detection thresholds, which require only awareness of some sound.

Speech threshold measures are most commonly used to verify pure tone sensitivity in the frequency range of 500 to 4000 Hz. The relationship between sensitivity for pure tones and for speech, however, varies with the type of measure—speech awareness threshold or spondee threshold—used. The sound pressure level at which speech can be detected on 50 percent of the trials (8 dB SPL) corresponds very closely to the average SPL needed for detection of tones in the 500 to 4000 Hz range (8.6 dB SPL). However, the average threshold for the higher level function (identification) is significantly higher: 20 dB SPL. As Figure 10–2 shows, detection and identification accuracy grow very quickly with increasing intensity on both tasks. Most clinical speech tests require a higher level of processing than detection; therefore, 20 dB SPL has been established as the norm for audiometric zero in defining the intensity at which speech signals are presented through earphones. The ST (in dB HL) should correspond to the pure tone average at 500, 1000,

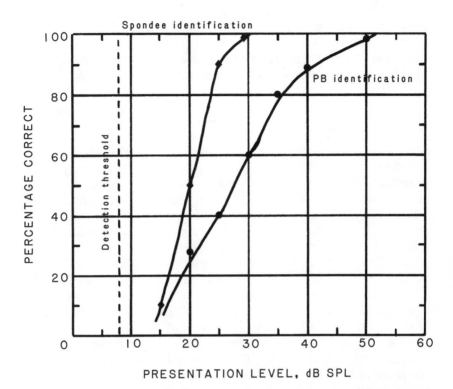

Figure 10-2. Performance-intensity function for detection (a) and identification (b) of spondee words. Note very steep growth of performance in each case. 50 percent detection is reached at about 8 dB SPL, but 20 dB SPL is needed for 50 percent identification of the speech stimuli.

and 2000 Hz within a range of +6 to −8 dB. Some examples of this relationship are shown here.

Pure Tone Average	Expected ST	Expected SAT
0 dB HL	−8 to +6 dB HL	−20 to −6 dB
25	17 to 31	5 to 9
40	32 to 46	20 to 34
67	59 to 73	47 to 61

What does it mean if the ST fails to agree with the pure tone average? Several explanations—some technical and some pathological—are possible.

First, output calibration may be inaccurate for the pure tones or the speech circuits on the audiometer. Second, some arithmetic error may have been made in calculating the PTA. Third, and closely related to arithmetic errors, is the influence of a steeply sloping or rising audiogram configuration when there is more than 20 dB difference between adjacent frequencies, as in the following example:

250 Hz	500	1000	2000	3000	4000	8000
10	15	25	70	75	70	85

In this case, the conventional PTA, derived from the mean of the thresholds at 500, 1000, and 2000 Hz, would be 37 dB. The spondee threshold, however, is likely to be considerably lower because of the good low frequency sensitivity. In cases such as these, the PTA is derived from the mean of the best two frequencies in the range (500 and 1000 Hz). These factors would be considered technical, or nonpathologic, causes of a PTA-ST discrepancy.

Striking PTA-ST discrepancies are often encountered in the audiometric data of persons with nonorganic auditory disorder. In this case, speech may be identified at a much lower level than pure tones; for example, a patient may have a PTA of 55 dB and an ST of 15 dB. What accounts for this discrepancy? Remember that speech is a complex acoustic signal, composed of many frequencies present more or less simultaneously. The perceived loudness of such a signal is greater than that of any component pure tone presented at the same intensity. When a listener attempts to feign impaired sensitivity, he or she usually finds it difficult to maintain thresholds for pure tones and for speech that relate to each other in the expected way. The speech material seems louder and thus is subject to less elevation than a pure tone. When spondee thresholds are lower than the pure tone average by more than 10 dB, the discrepancy should be examined more closely by looking into possible sources of error in the equipment and technique. Once external factors are ruled out, pure tone thresholds might be remeasured after reminding the patient to respond to the *very slightest* sound he or she can detect. An ascending approach to threshold is often useful in resolving these discrepancies. If the PTA-ST difference remains unacceptably large, special tests to investigate nonorganic disorder should be considered.

A second, and less common, basis of PTA-ST discrepancies can occur when retrocochlear auditory disorder is present. In this case, the spondee threshold may be *higher* than predicted by pure tone sensitivity because of the great speech distortion that such disorders can produce. Again, after ruling out possible external factors to account for this finding, special tests sensitive to retrocochlear disorders should be planned.

Word Identification Tests

Speech detection and identification thresholds give some indication of a minimal level at which a speech signal can convey information. If more insight into impairment for speech communication is desired, the clinician must turn to suprathreshold tests. Many such tests have been proposed over the years, ranging from the simple whispered voice test—the earliest form of speech "audiometry"— through closed set discrimination tests, to more complex sentence and paragraph comprehension tests. Only a few, however, have remained in widespread clinical use.

Description of Materials

Until recently, the speech materials used for suprathreshold tests in the majority of North American audiology clinics were monosyllabic words. These lists of words (50 per list) had been selected to satisfy several criteria, most notable of which was a phonemic distribution equivalent to that found in ordinary spoken English. For example, if /s/ accounted for 27 percent of all phonemes in a sample of running speech, /s/ would appear within the lists with 27 percent frequency as well. The materials developed in this way came to be known as *phonemically balanced* or *PB* word lists. One such list, taken from the Northwestern Auditory Test No. 6 (NU-6) is presented in Table 10-2. Other lists still in widespread use were developed at the Central Institute for the Deaf (CID W-22) and the Harvard Psychoacoustic Laboratory (PAL PB-50). All were designed with the common objectives of phonemic balance, word familiarity, and equivalent word difficulty among lists. One version of the PAL list was recorded by Rush Hughes, a speaker whose rapid, clipped midwestern pronunciation of the stimulus words made them exceptionally difficult to identify, even for listeners with normal hearing. A patient's measured word identification in quiet can be influenced by a number of external factors, including the types of materials and speaker, the intensity at which he or she is tested, and the variables of interest (i.e., a patient's site of disorder and audiometric configuration and severity).

Table 10-2.   Northwestern University Auditory Test Number 6

laud	love
boat	sure
pool	knock
nag	choice
limb	hash
shout	lot
sub	raid
vine	hurl
dime	moon
goose	page
whip	yes
tough	reach
puff	king
keen	home
death	rag
sell	which
take	week
fall	size
raise	mode
third	bean
gap	tip
fat	chalk
met	jail
jar	burn
door	kite

Clinical Applications

Traditionally, PB words are presented following a carrier phrase (i.e., "Say the word . . .") at a level 30 to 40 dB above the spondee threshold or the pure tone average. The choice of this level criterion arose from the observation that maximum word identification scores (sometimes called *PB-max*) are usually achieved by 30 dB SL re: ST *in normally hearing subjects*. Therefore, routine use of the 30 dB SL criterion implicitly assumes that the slope (rise to maximum) of the performance-intensity function is essentially the same in all patients. That assumption is probably valid for patients with conductive impairments, in which signal attenuation is the only problem, and for those with mild cochlear-based impairments. It can lead to error, however, when applied to patients with precipitously sloping high frequency impairment, those with moderate to severe impairment, and those with retrocochlear disorders. For example, the ST of a patient whose audiogram is shown in Figure 10-3 will reflect the normal sensitivity through 1000 Hz and fall in the 5 to 10 dB HL range. A word list presented 30 dB higher, at 40 dB HL (60 dB SPL), will underestimate that listener's word identification

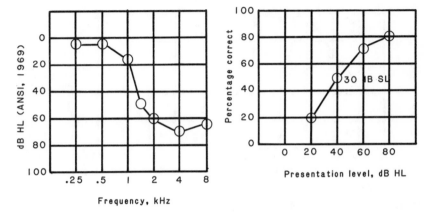

Figure 10–3. Audiometric data of a patient with a steeply sloping high frequency sensorineural impairment. The spondee threshold reflects the patient's good low frequency sensitivity, but word identification score is affected by the amount of high frequency information available to the listener.

ability because high frequency acoustic cues to consonant identity would be largely inaudible. Word identification improves at higher presentation levels as more acoustic information becomes available. By contrast, a patient with a flat audiometric configuration may experience severe loudness discomfort for speech presented 30 to 40 dB above his or her threshold, with a corresponding reduction in identification score. Here again the listener's maximum performance would be estimated incorrectly. In each of these cases, measuring word identification performance at a single intensity would lead to errors in interpretation because the location of that point on the performance-intensity function would be unknown. Similarly, if a patient's word identification has been measured at a single intensity, it cannot be described as "PB-max" if it is less than 100 percent, because "maximum" implies a comparison with other values.

Performance-Intensity Functions

In 1971 Jerger and Jerger described performance-intensity functions using the PAL PB-50 word lists (now called PI-PB functions) in patients with cochlear and retrocochlear eighth nerve disorder. They found that patients with retrocochlear disorders frequently displayed *reduced* word identification accuracy at stimulus presentation levels *higher* than that needed to achieve PB-max. This phenomenon, designated *"rollover,"* could be observed at signal levels of 100 to 110 dB SPL. Figure 10–4 presents a normal performance-intensity function contrasted with one showing rollover. Jerger and

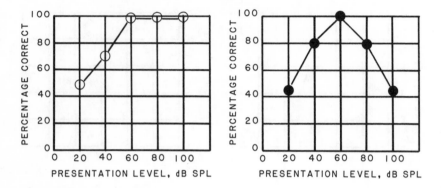

Figure 10-4. Performance-intensity functions for PB word materials. The function with open circles shows normal performance in which maximum performance does not decline with further increases in stimulus presentation level. The function with closed circles illustrates the "rollover" phenomenon in which word recognition is severely reduced at high intensity levels. Note that PB max is normal at 30 dB SPL in both functions.

Jerger recommended that clinical use of PB word lists not be limited to testing at a single intensity level, but that PI-PB functions be generated, if not routinely, at least in cases in which retrocochlear auditory disorder is a possibility. Later work demonstrated that the rollover phenomenon is not found exclusively in patients with eighth nerve disorder, nor do all such patients demonstrate rollover. Rather, it is closely linked to the presence or absence of the acoustic reflex (Hannley and Jerger, 1981) and has also been described among patients with facial nerve disorders (Borg and Zakrisson, 1973; McCandless and Schumacher, 1979), poststapedectomy patients (McCandless and Goering, 1974), and, most recently, normal listeners (Dorman, Cedar, Hannley, Leek, and Lindholm, in press). In each of these groups, absence of the acoustic reflex was associated with rollover in the majority of subjects. The abnormally low word identification scores at high SPL has been attributed to failure of the high pass filtering action provided by the acoustic reflex, permitting an unusually great amount of low frequency energy to enter the cochlea.

Procedural Issues in Speech Audiometry

When speech audiometry was being developed as a tool, a great deal of attention was devoted to procedural details that might influence the outcome of the test. Extensive studies were completed on ascending versus descending methods of speech threshold approximation, the use of 2 or 5 dB steps in bracketing threshold, and the advisability of testing patients with half-lists of 25 PB words rather than the full 50 word lists. Most clinicians now agree that thresholds can be measured validly using either an ascending or descending approach and that the difference in thresholds obtained with the two methods are so slight that the size of the increment is also not critical. This is especially true because the pure tone thresholds with which ST is compared are routinely established using 5 dB step sizes. In most patients, the slight differences in word identification scores obtained using half versus full lists are made insignificant by the differences in testing time.

Perhaps the most significant procedural debate lies in the question of whether to perform speech audiometry using prerecorded materials or whether to use the technique known as *monitored live voice* (MLV). Clinicians are rarely neutral on this issue but, as with many other controversies, advantages and disadvantages of each technique can be described. There are situations in which MLV is the technique of choice, and there are also times when recorded materials are preferable. Certainly no clinical facility should be limited to one method alone. An understanding of the strengths and weaknesses of each method will help the clinician make an informed choice when designing a test strategy.

The most important advantage of MLV speech audiometry is its *flexibility*. That is, stimuli can be presented at a pace that is appropriate for each patient; the standard 4 second response interval found on most prerecorded tests may be tediously long for a young patient who encounters no difficulty in responding to the stimuli, but it may cause an older listener to feel rushed in his or her responses. An additional advantage is that threshold testing can present only those spondee words that a patient is able to identify consistently during a training period; this advantage is not true of prerecorded lists. Some clinicians have noted that use of the MLV technique reinforces the patient's impression that the clinician is in active control of the test situation. On the other hand, speech materials presented with MLV are subject to differences related to speaker gender, regional differences in word pronunciation, speed of presentation, vocal quality, and fundamental frequency. These differences can change a listener's performance, leading to the false impression that word identification has improved or worsened. Moreover, a clinician who is attempting to read a word list, monitor his or her voice on the audiometer's VU meter to achieve some measure of inter-item consistency, and record the patient's responses—all of this simultaneously—not only may give the impression of not being in complete control of the test situation, but also is limited in the amount of patient observation he or she is able to carry out.

The use of prerecorded materials offers the important advantages of *stability, consistency,* and *test-retest reliability.* When the question of the stability of a patient's hearing impairment arises, it is important to be able to duplicate as nearly as possible test conditions from one test session to the next. A taped NU-6 word identification test administered at 80 dB SPL through TDH-39 earphones will have the same acoustic properties in Cleveland, Ohio, one year as it does in San Francisco, California, the next year, regardless of who is operating the audiometer. Unlike MLV, presentation of taped word lists does not require that the clinician be seated in a sound-treated room to prevent ambient noise from interfering with the test. In addition, professional recording techniques are able to minimize intensity variations on words within the lists. With increasing availability of digital recordings on compact disks, even the slight time-related deterioration of tape recordings will be a problem of the past. The disadvantage of prerecorded lists is that, inevitably, they require more testing time, owing to the set interstimulus intervals and identification messages at the head of each list. They cannot be used for testing an individual's auditory-visual processing in the same way that monitored live voice can, and, unless the clinic possesses copies of all taped speech materials, selection of materials that are appropriate for the patient's language level is limited. Thus, prerecorded materials are of limited flexibility but excel in reliability.

Limitations of Monosyllabic Word Lists

Monosyllabic word lists have several drawbacks as clinical materials. First, they contain words that may be unfamiliar (and thus are more difficult to identify) to many listeners: words such as *scythe* (PAL PB-50), *awe* (NU-6), and *mew* (W-22). Why is this a problem? In responding to the traditional PB word lists, listeners quickly perceive that the components of a word list are all "real" words rather than nonsense syllables; their error responses, therefore, may be shaped more by linguistic constraints than by their actual perception in making a response. Hence, a response of "side" or "size" to the stimulus word *scythe* may reflect a subject's unfamiliarity with the stimulus word, rather than a phonemic misperception. Second, word identification tests are scored using a binary system: a response is either correct or incorrect. Moreover, this binary system covers errors ranging from no response through substitution of one or more phones to addition of plural endings. This scoring procedure provides no information about patterns of phoneme confusions as they relate to an individual's sensitivity impairment; this information could then be useful in designing aural rehabilitation programs or in assessing amplification effectiveness. Third, word identification tests do not assess a patient's ability to use prosodic or contextual clues in processing speech for communication. Thus, word identification scores frequently are poor predictors of effective (i.e., social) hearing for speech. Moreover, there is no systemic pattern of word identification scores that would enable prediction or verification of sensitivity impairment. As Figure 10–5 shows, maximum word identification can remain at 90 to 100 percent with peripheral sensorineural impairment up to about 60 dB HL.

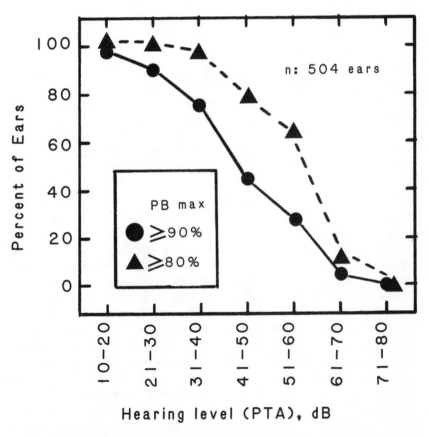

Figure 10–5. Maximum word recognition scores as a function of pure tone averages (500, 1000, 2000 Hz). Note that maximum scores can be normal with peripheral impairment up to about 60 dB HL.

SYNTHETIC SENTENCE IDENTIFICATION (SSI)

Description of Materials

As the previous sections have illustrated, isolated words and non-sense syllables have both strengths and weaknesses as materials for assessing hearing for speech. One major drawback to such tests is that it is difficult to draw inferences about how the stream of speech is processed. That is, ongoing speech is characterized by continuously changing intonation, loudness, and even speed over time. As actors and actresses know, these patterns supplement and some-times even override the information carried by words alone. Try saying these sentences aloud, stressing the italicized word:

> *What* do you want?
> What *do* you want?
> What do *you* want?
> What do you *want*?

Although each example contains the same words in the same order, the different intonation patterns would convey different meanings to a listener. Thus, sentences could be regarded as more versatile conveyers of information than any single word is.

Jerger, Speaks, and Trammell (1968) identified several disadvantages of using only single words for speech audiometry. First, single words cannot be manipulated to change intonation patterns over time. Second, single word tests are usually administered as part of an *open set* of stimuli; that is, when a subject hears a word, his or her response must be drawn from all the words in his or her response repertoire rather than from a limited set of alternatives. The open set method could also be described as an identification task. Third, when a subject repeats a word, the test score is influenced by the clinician's ability to perceive the response. The clinician, then, is forced into an open-set identification task similar to that of the subject. This can be a serious problem if the intelligibility of the patient's speech is degraded by an articulation disorder or a marked foreign accent, if the clinician has a hearing impairment, or if the speaker system used for monitoring is of poor quality.

Speaks and Jerger (1965) developed an alternative set of speech materials, which were intended to overcome some of the aforementioned problems. Rather than single words, they constructed "synthetic" sentences that followed specified rules of syntax and preserved intonation patterns found in conversational speech. The test sentences are shown in Table 10-3.

Table 10–3. Synthetic Sentences

Small boat with a picture has become.
Built the government with the force almost.
Go change your car color in red.
Forward march said the boy had a.
March around without a care in your.
That neighbor who said business is better.
Battle cry and be better than ever.
Down by the time is real enough.
Agree with him only to find out.
Women view men with green paper should.

Each sentence has seven words and from eight to ten syllables. They do not, you will notice, "make sense" although they can be read aloud with a normal intonation pattern. These sentences were described by Speaks and Jerger as "third-order approximations" to real (meaningful) sentences.

What is an approximation to a sentence? A sentence is usually defined as a word or group of words that expresses a complete thought, has a subject and a predicate, begins with a capital letter, and ends with appropriate punctuation. An approximation to a sentence is a group of words. If the words making up the "sentence" are completely unrelated to one another (i.e., drawn at random from a vocabulary list), the sentence is described as a "first-order approximation":

> Due his fit along sick near nearly.

The sentence could be made to sound more natural by making each word linguistically dependent on the word preceding it, as in

> Laugh long name my French women laugh.

Here, the "sentence" is constructed of a sequence of word pairs—laugh long; long name; name my; etc.—that would be linked together naturally in a meaningful sentence. This is called a "second-order approximation." A third-order approximation, then, could be developed by making every word (after the second) dependent on the two that precede it:

> Down by the time is real enough.

If the order of approximations were continued to a high enough level, a real sentence would eventually emerge.

Why go to this trouble to construct nonmeaningful sentences that only sound real? Speaks and Jerger wanted to avoid certain drawbacks that other open-set sentence tests had encountered, such as the biasing influence of the patient's vocabulary, information set, and linguistic experience.

The SSI is administered as a *closed-set* test; there are only 10 possible answers to each test item, the alternatives are always the same, and the patient has access to a list of the sentences from which he must select a response. This design largely neutralizes those biasing variables mentioned earlier because it creates a true *recognition* rather than an *identification* or *comprehension* task. The closed message set design also means that the patient need only identify a sentence by number when he or she hears it, practically eliminating the scoring variability arising from the clinician's perception or from imperfect intercom systems.

The performance-intensity function of synthetic sentences presented in quiet is extremely steep, similar to that for spondee words, and therefore it is even less efficient than PB words in reflecting subtle deficits in speech processing. Even patients with very poor word recognition achieve 90 to 100 percent correct sentence identification at sufficiently high intensities. This characteristic is not surprising, when we consider three attributes of the sentence materials: (1) the task is easier (i.e., closed-set recognition of sentences versus open-set identification of words); (2) the sentences are more redundant in the information they carry; and (3) the prosody (rhythm) of each sentence is distinctive. You can demonstrate the prosodic differences by replacing each syllable of the sentences by "da" as you read them aloud.

For these new materials to be clinically useful, it was clear to Speaks and Jerger that the task had to be made more difficult. The most effective means of increasing the difficulty proved to be adding a competing speech message to the sentences. A story about the life and times of Davy Crockett, a Texas frontiersman and folk hero, was read by the same talker who had recorded the sentences. Other forms of competition such as broad-band noise, speech babble or "cocktail party noise," speech played backward, and speech recorded by a different talker were evaluated. In each case, they had to be played at much higher levels than the sentences to provide as much competition as the same-talker discourse. Thus, the same-talker competition was more effective and more efficient than the other forms.

The relationship in intensity between the sentences and the background talking is called the *message-to-competition ratio* (MCR) and is analogous to the concept of signal-to-noise ratios used to describe nonspeech stimuli. A positive MCR means that the sentences are presented at a higher level than the competition; a negative MCR means that the competition is more intense. For example, + 10 MCR would indicate that the sentences were presented 10 dB higher than the competing story, whereas − 20 MCR would indicate that the sentences were 20 dB less intense than the competition. A series of experiments demonstrated to Speaks, Jerger, and Jerger (1966) that an MCR of 0 dB (sentences and competition equally intense) was most suitable for clinical evaluation, yielding scores equivalent to those derived from word identification tests in hearing impaired listeners.

Clinical Applications

The SSI materials have proved to be extremely versatile in assessing several levels of auditory function because so many of their parameters can be manipulated to meet different testing requirements. Presentation level can be varied to describe a performance-intensity function; similarly, the MCR can be varied for a performance-MCR function. The sentences can be filtered, time-compressed, or interrupted; the competing message can be played to the ear receiving the sentences or to the opposite ear for central auditory evaluation. In the basic assessment most attention is focused on the performance-intensity characteristics of the materials at 0 MCR as they relate to audiometric configuration and to the P-I function for PB words.

The 0 MCR function serves two roles in the basic assessment: (1) it is a cross-check on the audiogram configuration, and (2) it can indicate the presence of retrocochlear disorder. Both roles are fulfilled by evaluating the relationship between word recognition in quiet and sentence identification in competing speech as a function of audiogram configuration.

Many speech perception studies report that stop consonants and fricatives are poorly identified by hearing impaired listeners (Dorman and Hannley, 1984), particularly if the high frequencies (i.e., above 1500 Hz) are affected. Similarly, when PB word lists are low-pass filtered (high frequencies removed) and presented to normally hearing listeners, recognition scores are lowered; high-pass filtering does not produce the same deficit. By contrast, synthetic sentences become poorly intelligible with high-pass filtering but are relatively unaffected by low-pass filtering.

This being the case, differences in PB and SSI scores could reasonably be expected to vary with audiogram configuration. Jerger and Hayes (1977) defined patterns of PB-SSI relationships as a function of configuration in more than 3000 patients. When sloping high frequency loss exists on a peripheral basis, SSI scores are higher than the word recognition scores, as shown in Figure 10–6. The difference between the two maximum scores is called the *PB-SSI discrepancy*. The magnitude of such a discrepancy varies directly with the steepness of the audiometric slope and inversely with the frequency at which the slope begins. That is, the steeper the slope, the greater the discrepancy, and the lower the frequency at which the slope begins, the greater the discrepancy.

By contrast, a rising configuration will produce higher word recognition than SSI scores, especially at levels close to threshold. This relationship is shown in Figure 10–7. Again, the low frequency impairment interferes with reception of the relevant information in the sentences, just as high frequency impairment interferes with the consonant recognition on which the PB score depends.

When the audiogram is flat (i.e., <20 dB difference in thresholds for frequencies between 500 and 2000 Hz), little or no PB-SSI discrepancy is expected (Fig. 10–8). Impairment in the low frequencies affects sentence identification and impairment in the high frequencies affects word recognition. Table 10–4 summarizes the PB-SSI relationships expected from peripheral disorders of different configurations.

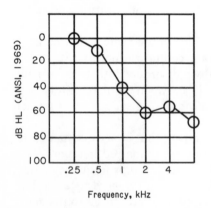
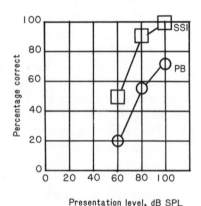

Figure 10–6. PB-SSI relationships expected when sloping high frequency audiometric configuration is present on a peripheral basis.

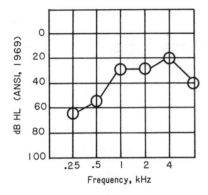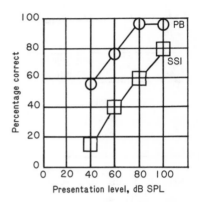

Figure 10-7. PB-SSI relationships expected when rising audiometric configuration is present on a peripheral basis.

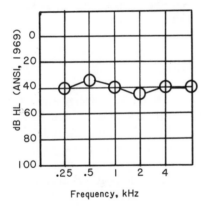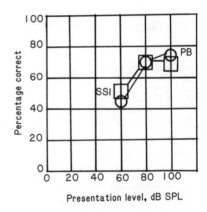

Figure 10-8. PB-SSI relationships expected when flat audiometric configuration is present on a peripheral basis.

Notice that when the impairment arises from a peripheral disorder, there is only one circumstance—a rising configuration—in which the SSI score is predicted to be lower than the word recognition score. If that configuration is *not* present to account for a PB-SSI discrepancy greater than 20 percent, a retrocochlear disorder should be suspected.

One aspect of the SSI procedure that has drawn some criticism is the fact that it requires reading competence on the part of the

Table 10–4.   PB-SSI Relationships with Various Audiogram Configurations

Audiogram Configuration	PB-SSI Relationship
Sloping	PB < SSI
Rising	PB > SSI
Flat	PB = SSI

patient. Thus, its use in younger subjects, in those with serious visual disturbances, or in those with reading disability of any sort would seem to be limited. In practice, however, the test can be administered and scored easily and with great success by having the listener simply repeat aloud all or part of the target sentence. That response mode is easily taught in a preliminary practice session in which the sentences are presented to the patient without the competing message. I have used the SSI successfully with patients belonging to each of the aforementioned categories.

MASKING IN SPEECH AUDIOMETRY

Chapter 7 was devoted to the principles of masking as they apply to pure tone stimuli. Whenever speech stimuli are presented at levels capable of producing cross-hearing, masking is also required. The rules governing the use of masking for speech signals are very similar to those used for pure tones:

1. *When to use masking:* Use masking if there is ≥ 40 dB difference between the air conduction of the test ear and the bone conduction of the nontest ear.
2. *What kind of masking to use:* Speech is a complex signal, composed of many frequencies. Therefore, a narrow band of noise would be capable of masking only certain parts of the speech signal and would be neither efficient nor effective. Speech is masked by using either broadband noise ("white noise") or a broad band of noise that has been filtered so that most of its energy corresponds to the spectrum of running speech. The latter type of masking is often referred to as "pink noise."
3. *How much masking to use:* The Hood plateau method of masking is not appropriate for determining masking level during speech audiometry. As a general rule, masking delivered to the nontest ear at a level 20 dB lower than the speech signal intensity will

be adequate. When the usual 40 dB interaural attenuation value for air conduction is considered, therefore, the noise in the non-test ear would be at least 20 dB higher than a crossed over speech signal from the test ear. Conversely, if cross-hearing took place, the noise level would be at least 60 dB lower than the signal in the test ear and would be unlikely to cause any significant change in performance.

STUDY QUESTIONS

1. Distinguish between extrinsic and intrinsic sources of redundancy in speech processing.
2. Why is "speech discrimination" not an accurate description of the PB word identification test?
3. What are some shortcomings of PB word materials? Of the SSI materials?
4. Why is the speech awareness threshold lower than the speech reception threshold?
5. What are the advantages of defining a performance-intensity function?

Chapter 11

Interpretation: Putting It All Together

The process of interpreting the meaning of a battery of auditory tests is, in some ways, analogous to assembling a jigsaw puzzle, the subject of which is unknown to you. The first step may be to locate the "edge pieces" to establish the framework and boundaries of the picture. Next, pieces with similar colors or patterns may be grouped together. As larger blocks of the puzzle come together, the subject of the picture becomes apparent; viewing the completed puzzle does not reveal the picture for the first time, but rather shows the finished details.

Similarly, interpretation of auditory test results is a dynamic process that evolves and is refined throughout the evaluation. In a very real sense, immittance audiometry provides the framework or the foundation of the battery with its multilevel information about auditory status. Cross-checks among similar tests are established along the way to develop the pattern of results and to meet the goals of the evaluation. As each new piece of information is acquired, it is compared to the existing set for consistency with the working hypotheses.

To illustrate this dynamic process of interpretation, the following case presentations are structured in the form of a dialogue that a clinician might have with himself or herself throughout the evaluation from the initial contact through the completion of the testing. For purposes of this demonstration, all equipment is known to be properly calibrated and in good working order.

CASE PRESENTATION 1

R. B. is a 15 year old male in apparently good health who responds readily to his name in the waiting room. His speech is well articulated and of appropriate loudness. He stands and walks with good balance. He does not appear to have any signs of neuromuscular disorder; both pinnae are present and well-formed; he does not wear a hearing aid or glasses. There is no apparent craniofacial abnormality.

Clinician. *Here is a person whose hearing for speech seems adequate. That could mean (1) he has normal hearing bilaterally; (2) he has normal hearing in one ear; or (3) his hearing impairment, if present bilaterally, is probably no worse than mild or is limited to a particular range of frequencies. His voice and articulation patterns sound normal. Thus, bilateral impairment, if present, probably is not long-standing or severe.*

There does not appear to be any suggestion of retrocochlear or central disorder in his physical appearance, movement, and balance. Similarly, there are no external signs to suggest congenital auditory disorder.

This is a young man: too young for military service or regular employment in a job that places him at risk for noise-induced hearing impairment. He may, however, have other, recreational sources of traumatic noise exposure.

The history reveals that R. B. has a chief complaint of decreased hearing in his right ear that he dates from a blow to the head suffered in an automobile accident two weeks ago. He comes to the clinic on a dual referral from an otolaryngologist and an attorney, who is pursuing the question of a personal injury settlement for R. B.

A blow to the head can cause a middle ear disorder such as tympanic membrane perforation or ossicular disruption. But it can also cause an sensorineural loss of any degree of severity, or a central disorder. I should also bear in mind that there may be a nonorganic component to the problem, since litigation is involved.

R. B. goes on to say that his hearing has always been good in both ears and that he passed all school hearing screening tests.

Hearing has been better than 25 to 30 dB HL, because this is the usual screening level. If immittance was used as a screening device, middle ear status must have been reasonably normal, as well.

Now, R. B. has a feeling of "stuffiness" in his right ear; he hears his own voice in his right ear, but it sounds "hollow, as if it's in a barrel."

He has the cochlear reserve to hear his own speech at the normal conversational intensities he is using, and it appears to be lateralized to his poorer ear. That sounds like a conductive problem. The stuffiness could be related to either middle ear or cochlear disorder.

Although he was "dizzy" and confused after the accident, R. B. did not lose consciousness and has had no true vertigo. There does seem to be a low roaring sound in the right ear, but it is hard to distinguish that from the "hollow" quality that is often present. He noticed the loss immediately after the accident, and it does not seem to have changed since then.

There was no significant brain concussion because he was not unconscious. The dysfunction appears to be stable rather than progressive or fluctuating. The sound in the right ear is a nonspecific sign.

Medical history is unremarkable, except for mild cases of measles and chickenpox as a preschooler. R. B. takes no medications regularly. His maternal grandfather has become slightly hearing impaired with advancing age and at present uses a hearing aid. Parents and siblings enjoy good health and hearing.

There do not appear to be any significant preexisting medical or familial genetic factors that might contribute to his problem.

R. B. has noticed since the accident that he now has difficulty hearing in the classroom sometimes, but not so much in the cafeteria: "I guess everyone's shouting in there, anyway." He notices that he seems to have trouble telling where sounds are coming from (i.e., localizing). This is a problem when he's playing basketball. Although these things bother him, he has no interest in considering a hearing aid.

If he has a unilateral hearing loss, he may not be seated in an optimum location in each classroom to hear the teachers. That will have to go into the management plan. His cafeteria experience sounds like "Willis's paracusis," a characteristic of conductive hearing loss. The background noise makes people speak more loudly to overcome its masking effect and maintain auditory feedback for monitoring their own speech (the Lombard effect). The effective signal-to-noise ratio is improved for R. B. by the louder voices coupled with the attenuating effects of a hearing loss on the noise. If it were a sensori-

neural loss, he'd probably report **more** *trouble in that situation. Difficulties in localization sound as if a unilateral hearing loss may exist, because auditory localization in space is highly dependent on the precise analysis of time and intensity differences at the two ears.*

R. B. attends a rock concert "occasionally," listens to his portable cassette player through earphones while riding his bicycle to and from school, uses power saws and drills in his wood shop class, is responsible for mowing the family's lawn with an electric mower once a week, and has ridden snowmobiles while visiting an uncle in Vermont. He has never used firearms, nor does he use ear protection.

There is a great potential for noise-induced hearing impairment in this part of the history. Counseling will have to include some discussion of ear protection, even if evidence of impairment does not appear in the audiometric data.

The history thus concluded, the clinician enters the testing area with the following information:

1. The goal of the evaluation is diagnostic; therefore, the tests chosen will be structured to search for a site of auditory disorder. Because the patient has had a head injury, this is particularly important. The co-referral from an attorney means that attention to all the appropriate cross-checks must be meticulous.

2. The chief complaint of the patient is that of hearing impairment and the effects it has had on his life in school and sports. The results of the tests will be most meaningful if related to those difficulties. The impairment, however, is not perceived by the patient to be sufficiently handicapping to consider a hearing aid.

3. There is evidence of a conductive impairment and further evidence that it may be unilateral, or at least asymmetrical.

The first set of tests will consist of the immittance battery. Both ear canals are inspected carefully with an otoscope and found to be clear of impacted cerumen, foreign bodies, and apparent infection. Both tympanic membranes can be seen and both appear to be intact with normal landmarks.

Good. This means I can test each ear with the immittance battery and get complete information. If the right ear looked abnormal in any way, I would not want to place the probe tip in it without first obtaining medical approval.

The left ear is tested first. The tympanogram, shown in Figure 11–1, has a base-peak compliance of 0.85 cc, with the middle ear pressure at -30 mm H_2O.

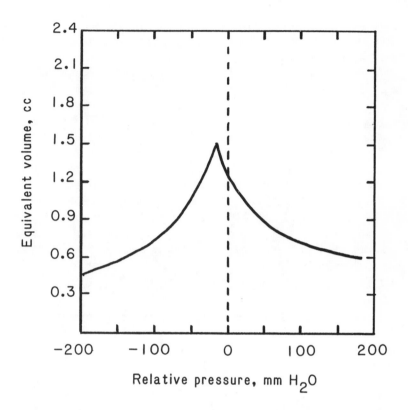

Figure 11-1. Tympanogram recorded from the left ear of subject R.B.

This is a Type A tympanogram. However, the slight negative pressure may affect reflex thresholds.

The right contralateral reflex thresholds (sound to right ear through earphone; probe still in left ear) are elevated at all frequencies beyond the equipment output limits of 115 dB HL. The left ipsilateral reflex thresholds (sound and probe left) are present at 105 dB SPL at 500 Hz, and at 90 to 95 dB SPL at the other frequencies.

The absence of RC reflexes could be a sign of conductive, sensorineural, or retrocochlear disorder. I will have to include bone conduction in the evaluation. The LI reflex is probably slightly elevated at 500 Hz due to the negative pressure; however, the fact that they are present indicates integrity of the afferent and efferent parts of the reflex arc on the left ear.

A seal is achieved with no difficulty in the right ear. R. B. remarks that he can just barely hear the "low humming sound" he heard when the probe was in the left ear.

Maintaining a seal at several pressures suggests that the tympanic membrane is intact and does not have some small unidentified perforation. The observation that the probe tone was barely audible suggests that a hearing impairment of about 65 dB HL exists for sounds in the region of 220 Hz, the probe tone frequency.

The tympanogram is quite deep, as shown in Figure 11–2, with a base-peak compliance of 1.72 cc. Middle ear pressure is in the region of 0 mm H_2O, although a peak cannot be defined.

This is a Type A_d tympanogram. Together with the absent RC reflexes, it suggests a middle ear disorder producing greatly reduced impedance (flaccidity), such as ossicular disruption. This is consistent with the history and with my working hypothesis. Also, if there is a nonorganic component, it is probably overlaid on a valid physical problem.

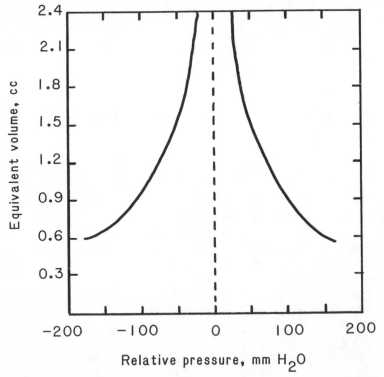

Figure 11–2. Tympanogram recorded from the right ear of subject R.B.

Acoustic reflexes cannot be observed at any frequency to ipsilateral or contralateral activators at equipment output limits.

This pattern of reflexes shows both a probe effect (LC and RI abnormal) and a sound effect (RC and RI abnormal), so this is an inverted-L pattern. This pattern is consistent with unilateral conductive impairment on the right. However, there could still be a central component associated with the head trauma, which is masked by the more peripheral disorder.

The reflex results are recorded on the audiogram. Pure tone air conduction thresholds are determined and are shown in Figure 11–3.

Sensitivity is normal for the left ear. The PTA is 8 dB. Masking will be required for air conduction on the right ear, because thresholds are at least 40 dB higher than the projected (by immittance results) bone conduction sensitivity for the left ear. The PTA on the right is 62 dB unmasked, and the configuration is flat.

This will be a good time to do a Stenger test to check for the presence of a nonorganic component. Even though there is evidence from immittance that a valid problem exists, there is no reason why thresholds might not be a little exaggerated, and that question will come up if the litigation proceeds.

The Stenger test at 1000 Hz shows changes in perceived location of the tone at the appropriate crossover intensity.

That's a negative Stenger result, indicating that the thresholds I've recorded are probably valid. This result gives me some assurance that a functional overlay to the problem is unlikely. That impression can be cross-checked when the PTA-ST comparison is made.

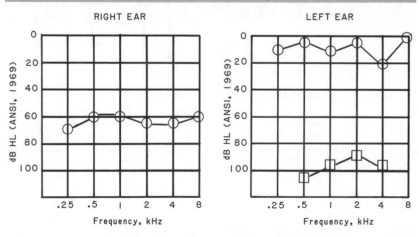

Figure 11–3. Unmasked pure tone air conduction thresholds of subject R.B. Note interaural asymmetry.

Narrow band noise is directed to the left ear for measuring masked air conduction thresholds on the right. A plateau was established at each frequency. Figure 11–4 displays the air conduction thresholds.

Is this masking adequate? At 1000 Hz, the threshold is 60 dB on the right and 10 dB on the left. Immittance results indicate that there is no air-bone gap on the left. Therefore, minimum adequate masking would be 10 (for AC on NTE) + 60 (for signal intensity) − 40 (for IA) − 10 (for BC on NTE) + 5 for the narrow band noise factor. That's 25 dB. My plateau extended from 30 to 60 dB masking, so according to the equation, it is adequate. The other frequencies can be assessed using the same process.

Bone conduction thresholds, as recorded from the right mastoid process, are determined without masking. All thresholds are within 0 to 10 dB HL.

Although there is evidence from the history and from immittance results that there is a conductive loss on the right ear, masking is necessary for bone conduction, because either ear could be producing these responses.

Bone conduction thresholds for the right ear remained essentially unchanged with narrow band masking levels of 30 to 60 dB HL directed to the left ear. As a cross-check, the occlusion index is

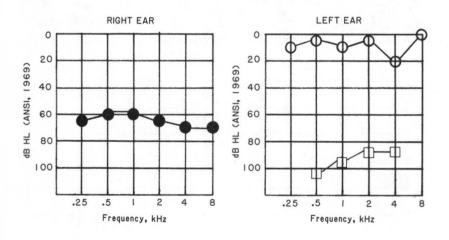

Figure 11–4. Masked pure tone audiograms of subject R.B.

determined for a 500 Hz tone; bone conduction thresholds are improved by 10 dB for the left ear when it is occluded, but are unchanged for the right ear. The completed pure tone audiograms appear in Figure 11–5.

This is a pure conductive impairment in the right ear because bone thresholds are within normal limits. The air-bone gap is consistently 55 to 60 dB—the maximum possible. That result, with the Type A_d tympanogram, the inverted-L reflex pattern, and the flat configuration, suggests ossicular disruption.

Spondee thresholds are determined: they are 5 dB on the left ear and 60 dB on the right, with 40 dB broad band masking directed to the left ear.

The ST agrees very well with the PTA in each ear. That reinforces my impression that there is no functional or nonorganic component.

Performance-intensity functions are described for the NU-6 phonemically balanced word lists and for SSI materials at 0 MCR. The functions are shown in Figure 11–6.

There is excellent word and sentence identification in both ears, although the maxima are reached at different intensities, reflecting the sensitivity loss in the right ear. SSI max is equivalent to PB max, and this is consistent with the flat configuration. There is no evidence of retrocochlear disorder in this test.

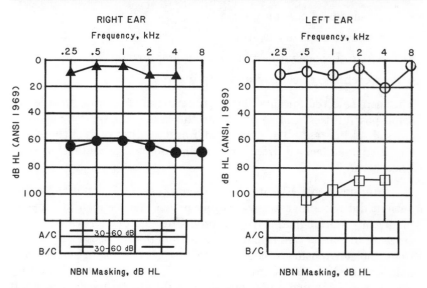

Figure 11–5. Completed pure tone audiogram of subject R.B.

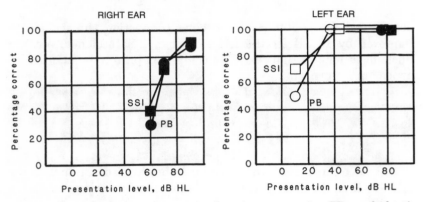

Figure 11-6. Performance-intensity functions comparing PB word identification and Synthetic Sentence Identification scores. The PB-SSI relationship is appropriate for audiometric configuration.

At the beginning of the evaluation, the clinician was faced with several diagnostic possibilities:

- Normal hearing bilaterally
- Conductive hearing impairment in one or both ears
- Mixed hearing impairment in one or both ears
- Sensorineural impairment in one or both ears
- Anacusis (dead ear) on the right
- Nonorganic auditory dysfunction
- Functional overlay to a true organic impairment
- Retrocochlear or central auditory disorder

The tests selected for this battery functioned efficiently to rule out some possibilities and to arrive at the same answer by means of cross-checking tests. The evidence for and against each of these possibilities (as derived from the total diagnostic contact) is outlined here.

Interview and History. The appearance and behavior of the patient did not suggest any vestibular disorder, congenital impairment, or neurological involvement. The history provided many clues as to conductive impairment, although the history of recreational noise exposure was extensive enough to raise a suspicion of noise-induced sensorineural component. The details of the auditory impairment sounded valid, but they could not be used to rule out nonorganic disorder. At the end of the interview, all eight possibilities were still being considered, but the evidence for conductive component was most prevalent.

Immittance Audiometry. This battery of tests was consistent in suggesting a middle ear disorder on the right. Therefore, unless a complex retrocochlear condition could account for the inverted-L pattern, the likelihood of a pure sensorineural impairment could be ruled out, but a mixed impairment was still possible. Similarly, the strong evidence of middle ear disorder tends to rule out normal sensitivity on the right.

Pure Tone Audiometry. Masked air conduction thresholds demonstrated a moderate sensitivity loss. This rules out anacusis and normal sensitivity. The normal masked bone conduction thresholds rule out the mixed loss hypothesis. The negative Stenger test provides evidence against the likelihood of a nonorganic disorder, and this was supported by bone conduction sensitivity within normal limits with air conduction sensitivity reduced. Such discrepancy is not typical of nonorganic auditory behavior, because most naive listeners are unaware of the physiological significance of the air-bone comparison. The conductive nature of the loss was cross-checked by the occlusion index.

Speech Audiometry. The spondee threshold was in good agreement with the pure tone average, providing more evidence that the impairment is not functional. The PB-SSI relationship is consistent with audiogram configuration; the slightly reduced maxima on the right ear can be accounted for by the severity of the impairment. Audiometer output limits (110 dB SPL) did not permit overcoming the attenuation created by the middle ear disorder and thus the scores recorded may not be representative of maximum performance. The slope of the PI function, however, is essentially identical to that of normal listeners. Retrocochlear signs in the form of PB and SSI rollover, or unexpectedly low SSI performance, were not present to suggest retrocochlear disorder.

All test results, therefore, were consistent with a moderate conductive hearing impairment in the right ear and normal sensitivity for pure tones and speech in the left ear. The patient returned to his physician for continued management, with recommendations for conscientious use of ear protection and for annual audiologic evaluations because of continuing occasions of traumatic noise exposure.

CASE PRESENTATION 2

H. K. is a 58 year old woman who responds readily to her name's being called in the waiting room. Her face is symmetrical when she smiles. She wears eyeglasses, but a hearing aid is not in evidence.

As she reaches out to shake hands, some swelling and twisting of the joints in her hands can be seen.

Clinician. *This patient has sensitivity for speech presented at normal conversational levels. There is no evidence of facial weakness or paralysis. If she is hearing impaired, vision becomes even more important, so the necessity of having regular eye care will have to be stressed. The joint swelling could be arthritis; because the large doses of aspirin that are used to treat arthritis can be ototoxic, that part of her history will require special attention.*

H. K. carries on a lively conversation in a pleasant, well-modulated voice on the way to the interview room. Once there, she states that she has come on the advice of her family physician to determine whether she should have a hearing aid.

There is no evidence in the speech patterns of congenital or long-standing bilateral impairment. Her chief complaint seems to be that of hearing loss and her evaluation objective is a hearing aid consultation.

H. K. states that she has noticed her hearing getting worse in both ears for about the last 5 years. A librarian by profession, she first noticed the problem when library patrons spoke softly or whispered when talking to her. When she attempts to converse with her family or friends in a restaurant or other noisy place, she seems to miss a lot of what is said. This makes her feel "silly" and left out sometimes.

This appears to be a slowly progressive loss, and there is no immediate history of occupational noise exposure. The difficulties in speech understanding, which suggest a sensorineural disorder, have already interfered with her social communicative abilities.

There is no history of vertigo or other forms of dysequilibrium, nor does H. K. report aural pain or fullness, headache, or facial weakness. She has experienced a high pitched ringing tinnitus bilaterally, which is continuous.

Accompanying symptoms are absent, except for the tinnitus. If the tinnitus is dose-related to the aspirin, part or all of the hearing impairment may be reversible as well.

The family history is negative for hearing impairment, with the exception of H. K.'s maternal grandmother, who developed a significant loss after a mastoid operation in her teen years. Other grandparents, aunts, uncles, cousins, parents, and siblings all hear normally.

The hearing impairment in the grandmother was apparently acquired and probably has no [genetic] relationship to the present hearing complaint.

The medical history reveals that H. K. enjoys good health at the present time, but that she is under a physician's care for rheumatoid arthritis, which she has had since her early 30s. She takes an average of 6 aspirin tablets per day and a steroid agent for this condition. The tinnitus does not seem to be related to taking the aspirin; it is present constantly and does not vary in its pitch or loudness. The only other medications used are multiple vitamins, taken daily. H. K. has had four pregnancies; all four children are alive and well. She has had no surgery or hospitalization other than for childbirth.

The medical history is significant for the arthritis condition but is otherwise unremarkable. There is already evidence of reduced mobility or dexterity of the fingers owing to arthritis; this must be taken into consideration when selecting a hearing aid, because it may be difficult to manipulate the very small batteries and controls found in certain hearing aids. The aspirin dosage is low enough that it is probably, as the patient believes, unrelated to the tinnitus. This impression is supported by the fact that the tinnitus does not seem to change between dosages.

H. K. is a nonsmoker and drinks an occasional cocktail or glass of wine on social occasions. She finds that communication is becoming more difficult, especially if there is noise in the background, and believes that although she seems to be relying on lipreading to a greater extent, it does not entirely compensate for her hearing difficulty.

H. K. is seriously concerned about the ways in which her social communication efficiency have been impaired. She is trying to develop compensatory mechanisms on her own, and thus she will probably be receptive to the idea of some aural rehabilitation. The social history is noncontributory.

Because this auditory problem has become noticeable only recently, H. K. has never had her hearing tested formally. She had a hearing screening test at a health fair in a shopping mall about 2 years ago and was advised at that time to have a more complete test and that she should consider a hearing aid. She did not follow up on that suggestion because she thought that the test results might have been inaccurate ("it was awfully noisy in there at the time") and because she did not want to be pressured into buying a hearing aid.

There is some evidence that hearing impairment might have been present as long as 2 years ago, although, as the patient observed, the test results may have been influenced by ambient noise.

The history being completed to both patient's and clinician's satisfaction, testing is begun. The clinician has learned the following:

1. The goal of the evaluation is twofold: first, to identify the nature and extent of hearing impairment; and second, to address the question of whether a hearing aid is indicated.

2. The chief complaint of the patient is hearing impairment that has interfered with social communication efficiency and has produced some psychological discomfort for her.

3. There is some evidence of sensorineural impairment, more likely to be bilateral than unilateral because the problem is described as a global one rather than being associated with either ear directly.

As usual, immittance audiometry is carried out as the first set of tests in the battery. Otoscopic inspection of the ear canals shows normal structures in each ear. There is a slight amount of cerumen in the left canal, but a portion of the tympanic membrane can be seen beyond the cerumen.

There is no indication that tympanometry should not be done. The small amount of cerumen should not interfere with any part of the battery.

The right ear is tested first. The tympanogram, shown in Figure 11–7, has a base-peak compliance of 0.42 cc, with the middle ear pressure at 0 mm.

This is a Type A tympanogram. Unless there is a problem along other parts of the auditory pathway, I should be able to observe some acoustic reflexes.

The left contralateral reflex thresholds (sound to left ear, probe in right) are within normal limits at all frequencies. The right ipsilateral thresholds (sound and probe right) are also 100 dB SPL or lower.

There is good evidence of normal middle ear function in this ear. Therefore, if there is a sensitivity impairment, it can be accounted for by a problem that lies beyond the middle ear. That being the case, bone conduction thresholds will not be necessary during the pure tone audiometry.

The two intact thresholds tell me also that the afferent part of the reflex pathway in this ear (represented by the RI reflex) is probably intact, as is the efferent part (represented by the RI and the LC reflexes).

The left ear (LC) is tested for reflex adaptation at 500 and 1000 Hz, at a level 10 dB higher (10 dB SL) than the reflex thresholds at

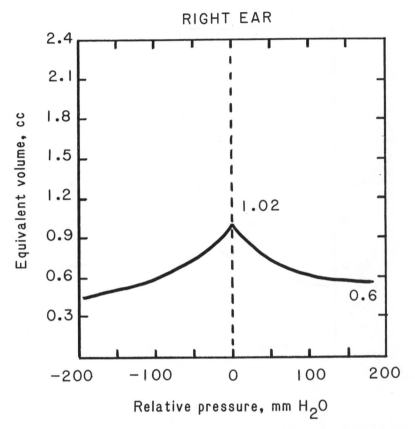

Figure 11-7. Tympanogram recorded from the right ear of subject H.K.

those frequencies. Reflex amplitude is maintained for 10 seconds at each frequency.

The absence of reflex adaptation does not rule out retrocochlear eighth nerve disorder, but it is strong evidence of cochlear disorder.

Static compliance on the left ear is 0.47 cc, with a middle ear pressure of 0 mm. Both contralateral (RC) and ipsilateral (LI) reflexes are present without adaptation at normal thresholds.

This is a Type A tympanogram [see Fig. 11-8]. Acoustic reflexes are normal and symmetrical with those measured from the left ear. There is less than 10 dB difference between the ipsilateral and contralateral reflex thresholds bilaterally. There is no evidence of retrocochlear eighth nerve dysfunction on the reflex adaptation test.

At this stage, the acoustic reflexes suggest symmetrical hearing bilaterally. Hearing impairment is probably no worse than about 60

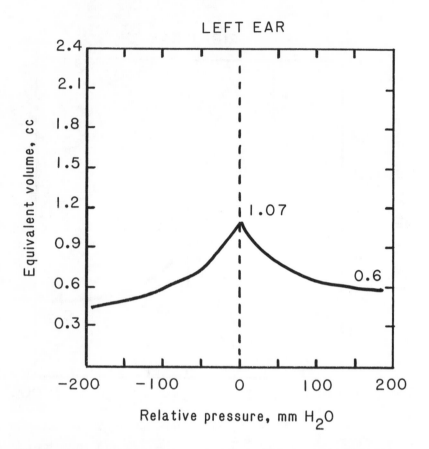

Figure 11–8. Tympanogram recorded from the left ear of subject H.K.

dB HL at any frequency, because reflex thresholds tend to become elevated with more severe impairments.

The reflex results are recorded on the audiogram. Pure tone air conduction thresholds are determined using a Hughson-Westlake procedure and are shown in Figure 11–9.

There is normal sensitivity through 500 Hz, declining to a mild loss at 1000 Hz and a moderate impairment for frequencies in the range of 2000 to 8000 Hz. Because the entire battery of immittance results was within normal limits on both ears, the loss can be assumed to be sensorineural and, therefore, bone conduction threshold measurement will not be necessary.

The PTA will have to be based on an average of the best two frequencies because the slope into the high frequencies is greater than 20 dB per octave. Therefore, the PTA is 12 dB in the right ear and 15 dB in the left ear.

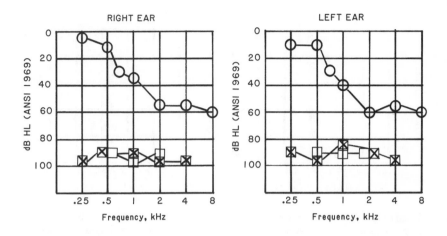

Figure 11–9. Pure tone air conduction thresholds of subject H.K.

Spondee thresholds are determined; they are 15 dB in each ear. *The ST agrees well with the PTA; there is no asymmetry so far on the speech testing.*

The PAL PB-50 word lists are used to determine the performance-intensity functions for monosyllables. Phoneme identification errors are noted to involve mainly stop consonants and voiceless fricatives. Vowel identification was unimpaired at PB max; at lower levels, both consonant and vowel errors occurred. The SSI materials, presented with a 0 dB message-to-competition ratio (0 MCR), are used to complete the speech function. The functions are shown in Figure 11–10.

When the stimuli are played at normal conversational level (60 dB SPL), the right ear has slightly better performance, although word recognition is reduced bilaterally at that level. The performance improves with increased intensity bilaterally. This tells me two things: first, there is no evidence of rollover as a retrocochlear sign; and second, amplification of speech, at least through these earphones, helps in word recognition. That is a positive sign for predicting the success of a personal amplification system.

The pattern of phoneme identification errors is consistent with the audiometric configuration and gives an indication of areas that will need to receive attention during the hearing aid adjustment and rehabilitation phase.

The SSI results give me two important pieces of information: first, my impression that this is a peripheral rather than a retrocochlear disorder is confirmed by the PB-SSI relationship, which can be accounted for by the audiometric configuration. Second, H. K. is still

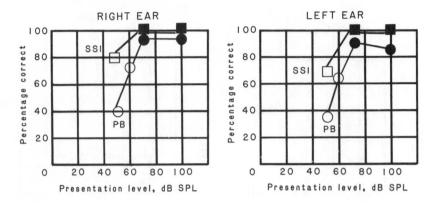

Figure 11-10. Performance-intensity functions of subject H.K., showing appropriate PB-SSI discrepancy for the sloping audiogram configuration.

able to identify stimuli presented at high levels against a background of competing speech; this too bodes well for amplification, although the test cannot be considered a direct analogue of understanding open-set speech in noise. I will feel comfortable in recommending hearing aid evaluation for this patient.

A dynamic range for loudness comfort and discomfort is determined, using conversational speech. Comfort level is 80 dB SPL on the left and 85 dB SPL on the right; the loudness discomfort level is at 105 dB SPL bilaterally.

There are reasonably wide dynamic ranges and provide more evidence that this patient is a good candidate for amplification. The levels are also in good agreement with the degree of sensitivity impairment that the pure tone audiogram shows. If the comfort levels were higher and the dynamic range wider, I might suspect either a hidden conductive or a retrocochlear disorder. All test results are far more indicative of sensorineural disorder of cochlear origin, however.

With only two exceptions, the test battery used for this patient was identical to that used to evaluate the previous patient (R. B.). Although the primary purposes of the two evaluations were different, many of the same tests could be applied, but their results were used in different ways. The pertinent information from each phase of the evaluation is presented here.

Interview and History. There was no indication from H. K.'s appearance and behavior that her primary problem was complicated by vestibular disorder, congenital disorders, or neurological involvement. The history revealed at least one possible contribution to an auditory disorder—long-term daily aspirin usage—although the symptoms did not seem to be temporally related. The description of the problem suggested sensorineural impairment, but H. R.'s voice and articulation patterns, being normal, did not suggest a severe deficit or one that had been present over a long period of time.

H. K. has already been troubled by the impact of her hearing impairment on her ability to communicate, and she has clearly indicated that she is interested in trying a hearing aid. Her motivation for amplification and aural rehabilitation, therefore, seems to be high.

Immittance Audiometry. All test results were consistent with normal middle ear function. Acoustic reflexes were present bilaterally and symmetrically, and this reduced the likelihood that severe (>80 dB HL) hearing impairment or a disorder affecting the eighth nerve or lower brain stem auditory structures was present. This information is important to the goal of the evaluation because it is necessary to ensure that, given preliminary medical approval, further medical referral is not indicated before proceeding with a course of hearing aid management and aural rehabilitation.

Pure Tone Audiometry. The areas of sensitivity impairment were defined by the pure tone audiogram, and this information will be of assistance in selecting aids to try during the hearing aid evaluation procedure. The progressively smaller differences in dB between auditory detection and acoustic reflex thresholds continue to support an impression of peripheral auditory disorder.

Speech Audiometry. The spondee thresholds were in good agreement with the pure tone average. This sign would not be expected with nonorganic disorder or, in certain cases, with central or retrocochlear disorders. The reasonably normal sensitivity for speech materials supports H. K.'s complaint that "speech is loud enough but not clear enough."

The speech functions were compatible with peripheral disorder; performance at high intensities showed potential benefit from amplification, both in quiet and with competing noise. These results, however, can only be considered approximations of H. K.'s potential to use a hearing aid for daily communication, because they represent performance while listening to limited types of materials through earphones under ideal circumstances. Another positive sign with respect to assessing the patient's suitability for hearing aid amplification was a reasonable tolerance range for speech in both ears.

All test results were consistent with sensorineural impairment on a peripheral basis. The test results also indicated a need for and potential benefit from hearing aid amplification. The patient was notified of these results and was given an appointment to return for the hearing aid evaluation. Her physician was sent a copy of the evaluation summary, recommendations, and a form for medical clearance to proceed with fitting for a hearing aid.

CASE PRESENTATION 3

K. L. is a 10 year old child who came with his mother to the clinic. He is reading a comic book in the waiting room and does not look up as you approach and call his name. K. L.'s mother instructs him to say "hello," which he does, in a quiet voice, before returning to his magazine. He does not wear glasses or a hearing aid; no external craniofacial or muscular abnormalities are apparent.

> **Clinician.** *This child does not respond to my voice at a normal conversational intensity, and his own voice is very quiet. At his age, a conductive impairment is not unlikely. There are no apparent signs of a syndrome associated with hearing impairment.*

On the way to the testing area, K. L.'s gait is noted to be normal, with no tendency to deviate in one direction or another. He does not respond to your question about his grade in school, asked on the way to the interview room. His mother, however, answers promptly.

> *It will be important to observe K. L. separately from his mother during the testing to assess his responses when not prompted by her; his failure to answer my question could have been as much a lack of opportunity as impaired hearing.*

Mrs. L. states that her son has failed a school hearing screening twice this year; his pediatrician has examined his ears, found them to be normal, and recommended complete hearing assessment and possible hearing aid evaluation. She goes on to state that K. L. is doing poorly in some school subjects and she attributes this to his "deafness." His teacher, however, does not think the youngster has a hearing problem and has recommended that he be seen by the school psychologist. Mrs. L. does not consider this an appropriate recommendation.

When asked directly, K. L. states that he is able to hear the teacher "sometimes" from his desk in the classroom. He does not maintain eye contact with you while responding, again in a quiet voice.

K. L. has not found it necessary to lipread as I speak to him at a normal conversational intensity; this is inconsistent with his behavior in the waiting room, although that may have been a simple case of shyness.

The history is accomplished quickly: K. L. is in excellent health, was born after a normal, full term pregnancy, had normal developmental milestones, is not under any medical care at present, and takes no medications. He has had no hospitalizations, no head trauma, and no chronic illnesses; he has had an isolated ear infection after an airplane trip at age 3. There is no family history of hearing impairment or of significant traumatic noise exposure other than to the usual household appliances.

This is a noncontributory history with respect to possible sources of the auditory complaint.

K. L. is asked whether he has noticed any noises in his ears. "Sometimes," he replies. The same answer is given to questions about dizziness or dysequilibrium, aural pain, or fullness. Further descriptions of these occasional symptoms are not forthcoming.

Mrs. L. is courteously but firmly directed to a waiting area with the assurance that she will be advised of the results of the assessment.

Otoscopic inspection of the ear canals show them to be clean, with no sign of infection or disease. No tympanic membrane perforations are apparent. Thus, immittance testing begins. Because K. L. reports that both ears are about the same, the right ear is tested first. The tympanogram is shown in Figure 11–11.

This is a Type A_S tympanogram because the base-peak compliance is less than 0.3 cc. Acoustic reflexes will tell whether this is significant.

Acoustic reflexes (LC and RI) are elicited without decay at thresholds ranging from 80 to 90 dB HL at frequencies in the range of 250 to 4000 Hz. The broad band noise threshold is 70 dB SPL.

If the Type A_S tympanogram represents some middle ear disorder, it is not severe enough to cause elevated reflex thresholds. I now know that hearing impairment, if present in this ear, is sensorineural rather than conductive and that sensitivity is probably no worse than moderately impaired.

The tympanogram from the left ear is shown in Figure 11–12.

This is a Type A tympanogram; base-peak compliance is within the normal range at 0.52 and middle ear pressure, inferred from the location of the tympanogram peak, is equal to ambient pressure. I would expect to see good reflexes in this ear, too.

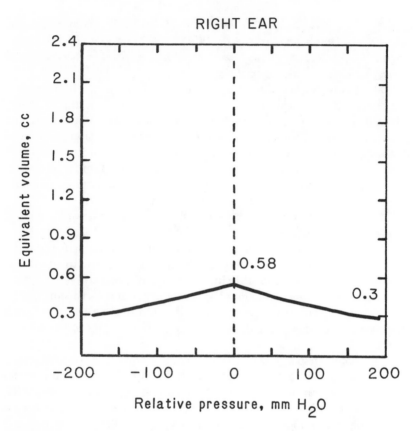

Figure 11-11. Tympanogram recorded from the right ear of subject K.L.

Acoustic reflexes are elicited with no decay to ipsilateral and contralateral tone activators at thresholds of 80 to 95 dB HL. *These reflex thresholds are symmetrical with those obtained with the probe in the right ear. Ipsilateral and contralateral thresholds are within 10 dB of each other. There is no evidence from acoustic reflexes of retrocochlear disorder or of middle ear disorder. Because there is no evidence of middle ear disorder on the immittance measures, my hypothesis of a conductive impairment as a basis for K. L.'s quiet speaking voice and inconsistent response to my voice does not seem likely. Perhaps there is a nonorganic component here.*

At this point the clinician must consider the following observations and data:

1. K. L. responded inconsistently to speech directed to him at a normal conversational intensity but did not appear to rely on lip-reading or other visual cues.

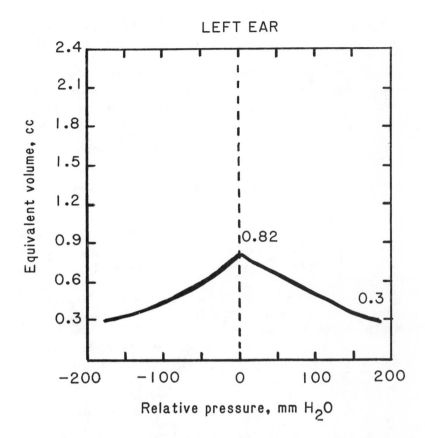

Figure 11-12. Tympanogram recorded from the left ear of subject K.L.

2. His vocal intensity is normal to soft and articulation patterns (from the limited speech sample available) appear to be normal.

3. There are no historical or physical factors that might be associated with hearing impairment.

4. Immittance audiometry demonstrated normal middle ear function; acoustic reflexes were present at normal thresholds, symmetrically, and without decay.

These observations would tend to rule out conductive disorder, but mild to moderate sensorineural impairment and nonorganic disorder continue to be possibilities.

Rather than beginning the behavioral tests with pure tone audiometry, spondee thresholds are approached next, ascending in 2 dB steps until K. L. repeats the first stimulus word at 15 dB HL on the right and at 20 dB HL on the left. With reinforcement for correct responses and urging to guess at the identity of the word, responses on a subsequent trial are obtained consistently at 10 dB HL in each ear.

K. L.'s sensitivity for spondee words is within normal limits; however, these words are highly redundant and familiar and I pressed him for responses. These STs do not rule out the possibility that there is a sensorineural impairment affecting the high frequencies. Before continuing with performance-intensity functions, pure tone audiometry is necessary.

K. L. is instructed to raise his hand as soon as he hears the tone in his ear, to keep his hand up as long as the tone is present in his ear and to lower his hand when the tone goes away. Twice during the test procedure the talkback level is set to 40 dB HL and he is asked whether he hears the tones. He responds "No." His voluntary (unmasked) air conduction audiograms are shown in Figure 11–13.

There are lots of inconsistencies here. First, K. L.'s pure tone "thresholds" are significantly higher than his spondee thresholds; in fact, they are higher at several frequencies than his acoustic reflex thresholds! This is not possible, because acoustic reflexes must be elicited at suprathreshold levels.

Second, although there is more than 60 dB difference between ears, there is no evidence of crossover in the form of a shadow curve response.

Third, he stated when asked that there was no difference between ears in hearing sensitivity. The pure tone audiogram, however, shows significant differences. Unfortunately, a Stenger test is not possible, because K. L. does not admit to normal sensitivity in one ear.

Fourth, he understood and responded to a question presented to him at a level corresponding to threshold on the left and well below threshold on the right.

Unmasked bone conduction sensitivity is measured, with the oscillator placed first on the right mastoid process and then on the left. The results are shown in Figure 11–14.

This, too, is inconsistent. The bone conduction thresholds are not in agreement with the air conduction on either ear; those measured from the right mastoid are higher than air conduction (A/C) on the left but show a large air-bone gap on the right, which is not supported by the results of immittance audiometry. Moreover, when the oscillator is placed on the left mastoid, thresholds are substantially different from those obtained with right mastoid placement. Because these are unmasked, the thresholds should be approximately the same, allowing for slight differences in positioning. So far, the preponderance of results suggest a nonorganic disorder.

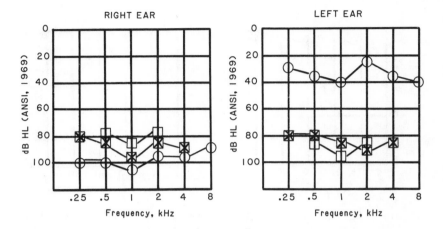

Figure 11–13. Voluntary unmasked air conduction thresholds of subject K.L.

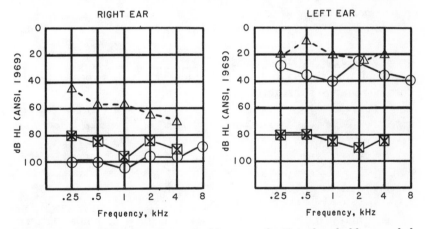

Figure 11–14. Voluntary unmasked bone conduction thresholds recorded from each mastoid; right ear "thresholds" indicate responses with the bone oscillator on the right mastoid process; left ear "thresholds" indicate responses with the bone oscillator on the left mastoid process.

K. L. is instructed to simply repeat the words that he hears. Monosyllable word lists are presented at 40, 60, and 100 dB SPL in each ear. The performance-intensity functions are shown in Figure 11–15.

These PI-PB functions are consistent with the better sensitivity suggested by the ST. The PB words are identified with 68 percent accuracy at a level only 10 dB higher than the admitted pure tone

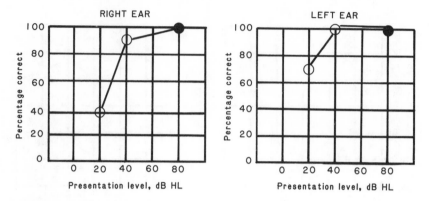

Figure 11–15. Performance-intensity functions for PB words of subject K.L. Note discrepancy between average voluntary pure tone detection thresholds (in Fig. 11–13) and low intensity word identification scores.

sensitivity on the left, and reach 100 percent at 60 dB SPL, a normal conversational intensity.

On the right, 40 percent identification accuracy is achieved at a level 58 dB lower than the admitted pure tone average, 88 percent accuracy is reached at 60 dB SPL.

When masking is directed to the left ear, K. L.'s vocal intensity does not change substantially.

If the hearing impairment in the right ear were valid, I would expect some increase in vocal intensity as K. L. attempted to maintain auditory feedback in the presence of noise. That is, the noise would prevent him from monitoring his own speech in his better ear. However, if he is able to continue self-monitoring in this right ear, masking noise on the left has no effect. This finding is called a negative Lombard effect.

The many inconsistencies in this patient's response patterns strongly suggest that the impairment is primarily nonorganic, although some slight organic basis has not been ruled out. The specific findings that lead to such a conclusion in each of the segments of the evaluation procedure are as follows:

History. According to the information provided by Mrs. L., her son has been in good health, with apparently normal hearing until this year, when he failed the routine school hearing screening test. Because his speech and language development has proceeded normally, and because he has passed all other hearing screening tests administered through the schools, the recent failure would suggest an acute or relatively sudden onset of the problem. However, there were no items in the history that would be associated with a sudden onset, and in fact K. L. did not describe any changes in his hearing to his parents or teacher, although the magnitude of the impairment he presented on pure tone testing would certainly have been noticeable to a 10 year old child.

It is possible that K. L.'s hearing had been affected by a middle ear disorder on the occasions of previous tests, but otoscopic examination by his pediatrician found no evidence of such a problem, and because the youngster had not been prone to recurrent otitis media at earlier ages, an isolated incident is less likely. Of possible significance is the surprising willingness of Mrs. L. and the pediatrician to accept the impairment and to use it to account for K. L.'s problems in school.

Immittance Audiometry. With the exception of a slightly shallow tympanogram on one ear, the results of these tests were consistent with normal middle ear function. The presence of normal acoustic reflexes in each ear does not indicate normal sensitivity, but it does provide an estimate of the upper limits of degree of impairment (i.e., no worse than about 65 dB HL). Lower reflex thresholds to broad band noise activators also suggest no more than mild impairment, because noise reflex thresholds increase almost monotonically with degree of pure tone impairment.

Pure Tone Audiometry. The voluntary pure tone thresholds are inconsistent with K. L.'s use of hearing for communication as observed during the history. Severe to profound impairment in the right ear is clearly impossible, because the reflex thresholds were themselves within normal limits. Cross-hearing does not occur at the appropriate levels, although there is greater than 40 dB difference between the air conduction on the right and the bone conduction (inferred from normal immittance results) on the left. Interaural differences in unmasked bone conduction thresholds are greater than can be accounted for on the basis of technical variables, such as placement of the oscillator, and there are unacceptably great discrepancies between air conduction and bone conduction sensitivity in each ear. That is, B/C is poorer at some frequencies than A/C on the left, and this is not theoretically possible; in the right ear, there appears to be an air-bone gap, yet the results of immittance audiometry clearly indicate that middle ear function is normal. Response inconsistencies in bracketing threshold are not consistent with sensorineural impairment, in which loudness recruitment usually ensures 100 percent response frequency to suprathreshold stimuli.

Speech Audiometry. Spondee thresholds are consistent with sensitivity in the 2 to 16 dB HL range (− 8 to + 6 dB is the acceptable area of pure tone–speech agreement) for at least two frequencies in the range of 500 to 2000 Hz. Performance-intensity functions for PB words show a normal slope, with words identified accurately far below admitted pure tone thresholds. There is a negative Lombard effect with masking noise to the better ear, demonstrating maintenance of adequate auditory feedback in the "poorer" ear.

Although the preponderance of data suggests that K.L.'s problem has a nonorganic basis, the possibility that his test behavior could be related to more subtle types of organic problems cannot be dismissed out of hand. For example, Berlin (1982) has found substantial numbers of individuals with severe to profound sensorineural impairment in the usual audiometric range of 250 to 8000 Hz who have intact sensitivity for frequencies in the range of 10,000 to 18,000 Hz. Many of these patients had been diagnosed as having a "functional" or nonorganic problem because their sensitivity for speech (and their speech production) was far better than might have been predicted on the basis of their pure tone audiograms. In this case, the presence of normal acoustic reflexes and the large discrepancies on bone conduction testing make that possibility less likely.

Reports have also been made of patients with temporal lobe disorders who show normal speech sensitivity with elevated pure tone thresholds (Jerger et al., 1969). In these patients, the temporal summation of loudness is so abnormal that pure tones presented with their usual duration of 500 to 1500 ms do not become perceptible to the patient until well above his or her "true" organic threshold. Here again, a pure tone–speech discrepancy would be seen, along with normal acoustic reflex thresholds. If a central basis for this recent auditory disorder is suspected, the child can be referred for an appropriate battery of tests. In the meantime, what information should be provided to Mrs. L., who is anxious to know the evaluation results and your recommendations?

I have found it most useful over the years to approach this situation on a positive note and to tell the understandably worried parent, "Good news! I have evidence today that [K.L.'s] hearing is probably pretty close to normal. I say 'probably pretty close to normal' because sometimes his *listening* is not very good, and that makes it difficult to define his exact level of *hearing*." When coupled with descriptions of positive behavior (e.g., sitting still for such a long time, repeating all the words nicely and clearly, taking so many tests), this approach has the advantage of not discrediting the school screening effort and, importantly, it does not imply motives of "faking" and "malingering" in the child that may result in more negative consequences when he leaves the test area. In most cases, I deliver this news to parent and child together so that the child learns (1) that you have recognized his good behavior and perceive him as a good person, but (2) that you are aware of the nature of his test behavior; (3) that it can be described objectively, without assigning blame or necessitating punishment; and (4) that there isn't anything really wrong with his hearing, as he may secretly fear. The child's ability to communicate efficiently at normal conversational levels should be stressed, if evidence to that effect is available. If more discussion of the significance of the screen failure is desired, it can be pointed out that many variables can affect a school screening test: excessive background noise, failure to understand the instructions, distractions, peer pressure, and so forth.

In the case of adult patients, it is necessary to proceed more cautiously, especially if legal action is involved. In that case, it is usually prudent to limit the posttest discussion to thanking the patient for coming in for the evaluation and assuring him or her that a full report of your findings will be sent to the designated persons. Confronting a patient with evidence of nonorganic disorder is rarely productive of anything other than hostility or defensiveness. It is important to bear in mind that malingering implies a conscious, deliberate fabrication of symptoms that the patient knows do not exist, for the purpose of secondary gain. Unless a patient admits to these elements—which rarely happens—you cannot know his or her motives.

CASE PRESENTATION 4

M. R. is a slightly stout 43 year old woman who turns immediately to greet you as you enter the waiting room. She does not wear eyeglasses or a hearing aid, and there are no immediately apparent craniofacial or neuromuscular abnormalities. Her handshake is firm as she looks you in the eye and smiles. You note that her smile is asymmetrical, showing a weakness on the left side, although the face is not completely paralyzed on that side.

Clinician. *The facial weakness is the most striking physical characteristic of this woman; I'll want to question her carefully about its onset, because facial nerve disorders can arise from a number of sources in the ear and nervous system.*

As you proceed into the interview room, allowing M. R. to precede you, you see that she seems a bit unsteady and reaches out to the wall to support herself. She laughingly refers to the way she "looks like [she's] had too much to drink" lately, although she rarely drinks alcohol.

So this gait disturbance is apparently of recent onset; I wonder if it's connected to the facial weakness?

M. R. states that she has been referred by a local otologist for diagnostic evaluation of a "nerve-type" hearing loss in her left ear. She first noticed the loss about a year ago when she found she was not able to understand speech over the telephone as clearly with the left ear as with the right. At that time she was recovering from a viral illness and thought she might have some "plugging up" of the ear as a result.

The patient is describing a unilateral hearing impairment that she has noticed only recently; this is a serious matter, considering the facial weakness (also on the left) and the dysequilibrium I noted. In combination, the three symptoms suggest retrocochlear disorder.

Within the last 3 months, M. R. reports, she has experienced dizziness "like the room is spinning and I'm going to fall." That sensation has been occurring more frequently and, as its onset is unpredictable, M. R. has stopped driving her car to work. The dizziness apparently is unrelated to body, head position and/or motion and usually does not cause nausea to the point of vomiting. The episodes last from 15 minutes to 2 hours.

M. R. has described a true rotary vertigo of the objective type. Episodic vertigo with hearing impairment can occur on either a cochlear or a retrocochlear basis, but the facial weakness would be more typical of retrocochlear disorder if, in fact, it is related to the other complaints.

After the first few episodes of vertigo, M. R. was examined by her family physician, who ordered laboratory tests and a skull x-ray. The x-ray results were normal, and the laboratory tests indicated "slightly low blood sugar." This was thought to be the cause of her dizziness. M. R. did not mention the hearing loss to the physician because "it didn't seem to be that big of a problem at that time." She has never experienced tinnitus.

M. R. noticed the facial weakness about 2 weeks ago, while applying makeup. She had not been ill, injured, or under unusual stress at the time. She subsequently consulted an otologist, who referred her to the present facility after examining her and testing her hearing with tuning forks. Special radiographic studies, including a computed tomographic (CT) scan, have also been ordered and will be completed tomorrow.

> *The facial weakness would appear to be broadly related in time to the other symptoms; there is no history that might lead me to associate the weakness with middle or outer ear infection, head trauma, or stress.*

With the exception of the otologist, M. R. is at present under no medical care. She takes an antivertigo medication as needed and finds it helpful. Medical history includes hospitalizations for a tonsillectomy and adenoidectomy at age 4; appendectomy at age 20; and gallbladder removal at age 41. Recovery from all surgeries was uncomplicated and she considers her health to be good.

There is no family history of hearing impairment; there have been no occasions of traumatic noise exposure in her occupation as a certified public accountant. Her chief leisure time activities include reading and participating in community little theater productions.

> *There appear to be no contributing factors to this patient's history before the onset of her present symptoms.*

When asked about the impact of the hearing problem on communication efficiency, M. R. replies that although she can hear very little with her left ear, she considers it a "minor inconvenience" to have to switch the telephone to her right ear rather than using the left ear, as she had been accustomed to doing. She finds that she has no trouble understanding people speak so long as there is not too much noise in the background. Of far greater concern to her is the facial weakness and the dysequilibrium.

> *This suggests that the hearing in the right ear is close to normal and thus social communication is affected very little.*

Immittance audiometry is used to begin the evaluation. The tympanograms recorded from each ear are shown in Figure 11–16.

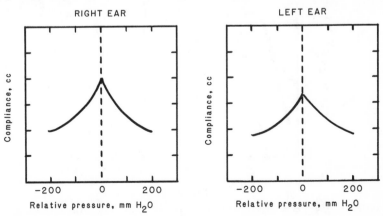

Figure 11–16. Tympanograms recorded from each ear of subject M.R.

> *Static compliance, middle ear pressure, and pressure-compliance functions are all within normal limits. I would not expect a middle ear disorder to interfere with my ability to elicit and observe acoustic reflexes.*

With the probe in the right ear, contralateral acoustic reflexes from the left ear are absent at equipment limits of 115 dB HL for activators of 1000 to 4000 Hz. At 500 Hz a reflex can be observed at 95 dB HL. Reflex decay is tested at that frequency, with the result shown in Figure 11–17. The right ipsilateral reflexes are elicited at normal thresholds.

> *The presence of the normal RI reflex confirms normal middle ear function on the right; it also assures me that both the afferent and the efferent parts of the reflex are functioning properly on the right. The absent LC reflex could be due to severe to profound hearing impairment (as the patient described), to a retrocochlear eighth nerve disorder, to an isolated abnormality of the LC pathways in the brain stem, or to a middle ear disorder on the right that has attenuated the activator tone. However, positive reflex decay at one frequency is far more suggestive of a retrocochlear disorder. The reflex pattern will become clear when I test the other ear.*

With the probe in the left ear, the right contralateral reflex is present, but at very low amplitude and at thresholds that are elevated at some frequencies. The left ipsilateral reflex is absent at equipment limits for all test frequencies. Reflex decay cannot be measured on the RC because of the elevated threshold and equipment output limits.

> *This pattern is basically diagonal, although a case could be made for calling it an inverted-L on the basis of the two elevated RC*

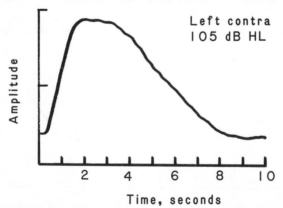

Figure 11–17. Acoustic reflex decay test for the left contralateral reflex. Note decline in reflex amplitude during the 10-second stimulation period.

thresholds. The low amplitude reflex may be related to the apparent seventh nerve disorder and facial weakness. Although it is fairly certain that this is a sensorineural impairment, bone conduction threshold measurement will be necessary to rule out a co-existing middle ear disorder on the left.

Unmasked air conduction thresholds are obtained without difficulty and are shown in Figure 11–18. M. R. reports that the sound in the left ear sounds "different—not as clear" as that in the right.

Here is an interesting observation. M. R. told me that there was almost no hearing in the left ear, yet her pure tone sensitivity is no more than mildly to moderately impaired. She has also described a qualitative difference between the tones in the two ears. Both of these signs are highly suggestive of retrocochlear involvement.

Masking will be necessary only at 4000 and 8000 Hz, because at lower frequencies there is less than 40 dB difference between the left ear's A/C and the right ear's B/C, as inferred from the immittance studies.

A pure tone Stenger test is attempted at 1000 Hz. It is negative until the patient reports that she hears the two different sounds— one in each ear—with the tone in the right ear remaining more distinct. Air conduction thresholds on the left are unchanged by narrow band masking directed to the right ear.

The failure to form a midline image of the two tones supports the patient's description of the qualitative difference and implies a problem in two-ear interaction.

Bone conduction thresholds are measured in the left ear. They approximate the air conduction sensitivity, with no significant air-

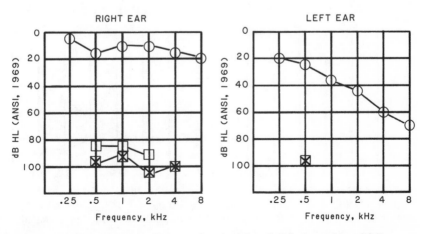

Figure 11–18. Unmasked air conduction thresholds for subject M.R.

bone gap. The completed pure tone audiograms are presented in Figure 11-19.

Now I know that I cannot account for the abnormal acoustic reflexes on the left by means of even a slight middle ear disorder; nor can they be accounted for by severe hearing impairment. The diagonal pattern appears to be related to retrocochlear disorder at the level of the eighth nerve or cochlear nucleus.

The spondee thresholds are 5 dB on the right and 25 dB HL on the left. The performance-intensity functions for PB words and for synthetic sentences at 0 MCR are shown in Figure 11-20.

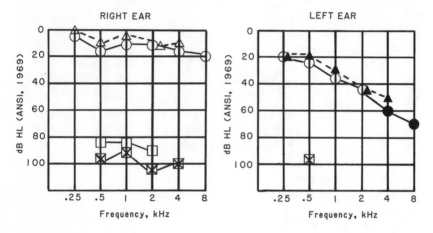

Figure 11-19. Completed pure tone audiograms for subject M.R.

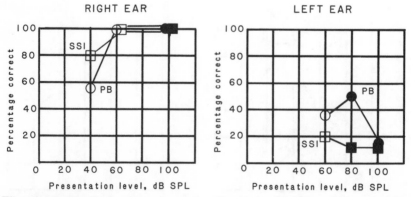

Figure 11-20. Performance-intensity functions for PB words and SSI materials for subject M.R. Note low PB max, rollover, and inappropriate PB-SSI discrepancy on the left ear.

The right ear shows good word identification at all intensities; there is no evidence of rollover. The left ear has maximum word identification far poorer than I would expect on the basis of the pure tone audiogram, and rollover appears as well. These findings are also consistent with the patient's description of "almost no hearing" on the left, because she would tend to equate her auditory function with her ability to understand speech. The low PB max is a retrocochlear sign, and the rollover might have been predicted by the predominantly absent acoustic reflexes in this ear.

The SSI functions are normal in the right ear but are certainly abnormal on the left. For one thing, the SSI max is lower than the PB max, and this is not consistent with the audiogram configuration. There is also some slight rollover, but the maximum was so low that identification accuracy could not get much lower. I know that she understands the task, however, because of the good performance with the same materials on the right and because she was able to identify the sentences with 90 percent accuracy at +10 MCR on the left. Therefore, these results are also consistent with retrocochlear auditory dysfunction.

The suspicion of retrocochlear disorder was in the front of the clinician's mind almost from the first moment of contact with the patient, but other diagnostic possibilities were not discarded without the appropriate cross-checking evidence. "Textbook cases" such as this one appear only infrequently in actual clinical practice, but for purposes of illustration, the patterns of interview, observation, and test results that confirmed that suspicion are summarized here.

Interview and History. Facial weakness or paralysis that is unrelated to head trauma, ear disease, or diabetes always indicates the possibility of retrocochlear or central auditory disorder until proved otherwise. In this patient's case, the facial weakness was not an isolated symptom but was also related in time to vertigo and unilateral hearing impairment. Moreover, the symptoms did not appear simultaneously, as they might with head trauma or vascular insufficiency (a "small stroke"), but sequentially—first hearing loss, then dysequilibrium, now facial weakness—in a way that suggests progression of a disorder. It is important to emphasize, however, that the symptoms reported by this patient may also be completely unrelated to each other. The information gathered from the interview and history should lead to hypotheses, not to conclusions.

Immittance Audiometry. The possibility of a conductive component could not be ruled out by this set of tests: unilateral middle ear disorders will produce inverted-L reflex patterns with Type A tympanograms and normal static compliance. The presence of reflex decay, however, is strongly suggestive of eighth nerve disorder, and an inverted-L pattern produced by a combination of a diagonal and a vertical pattern is not unrealistic, considering the evidence of facial nerve disorder in this patient.

Pure Tone Audiometry. The pure tone results rule out normal hearing sensitivity. In an attempt to account for the abnormal acoustic reflexes in the left ear, conductive impairement is ruled out by the lack of an air-bone gap and a normal occlusion index; severe to profound sensitivity impairment above 500 Hz (in the area of the absent acoustic reflexes) is ruled out by thresholds no higher than 60 dB HL.

Unilateral sensorineural impairment is generally atypical of purely cochlear disorders without some clearly related event in the history; it does not, however, exclude co-existing cochlear and retrocochlear disorders. The undetected contribution of a nonorganic component is difficult to rule out absolutely in behavioral testing, because it is the patient who decides when to respond to the stimuli. In this case, the negative Stenger test results, combined with the patient's description of her subjective auditory experience and her lack of a clear motive for giving false responses, make a nonorganic overlay an unlikely alternative.

Speech Audiometry. The close agreement between pure tone averages and spondee thresholds provides another reassurance that the voluntary pure tone thresholds are probably valid. Very poor word and sentence identification on the left lends credence to the patient's earlier report that she hears very poorly with this ear and considers it functionally deaf. The PB-SSI discrepancy cannot be accounted for by the audiometric configuration, suggesting retrocochlear disorder. The presence of rollover in both performance-intensity functions on the left ear is another retrocochlear sign and is consistent with the absent acoustic reflexes.

At this point, the basic assessment procedure is concluded. Because of the strong evidence of retrocochlear disorder, further special testing—beyond the scope of this book—is indicated. In some clinics, special "site of lesion" tests would be planned, including threshold and suprathreshold tone decay, short increment sensitivity index (SISI), loudness balance procedures, Bekesy audiometry, and other sensitized speech tests. Speaking as a clinician, however, my own strategy would be to bypass these behavioral tests and (if the necessary equipment were available) go directly to the most powerful auditory test of retrocochlear eighth nerve and brain stem integrity, auditory brain stem response audiometry (ABR). The choice of advanced diagnostic tests, as well as their interpretation within the test battery, is most efficiently governed by a knowledge of the principles of clinical decision analysis (CDA). This topic will be considered briefly in the following section.

CLINICAL DECISION ANALYSIS

The previous case studies have demonstrated the process of clinical interpretation as it might evolve with an experienced clinician. This process depends heavily on recognition of patterns in the patient's appearance and behavior, in the details of the history, and in the combined results of auditory tests. In the ideal situation, the patterns are clear, leading unambiguously to one conclusion. Far more often, however, the pattern is not clear because of mixed results that could be interpreted in more than one way. In such cases, an understanding of the principles of clinical decision analysis is invaluable.

As defined by Turner and Nielson (1984), clinical decision analysis is a "systematic approach to decision making under conditions of uncertainty" (p. 125). Interpretation of clinical data ultimately involves a series of decisions: decisions as to the nature of an auditory disorder; decisions about management alternatives; and decisions about the significance of certain test results within the context of a test battery. Each of these decisions can, in the most simplistic sense, be either correct or incorrect. Each incorrect decision carries its own price, just as there is some benefit associated with each correct decision. The uncertainty arises from the fact that few diagnostic tests of any kind are without error in identifying disease or dysfunction.

The Decision Matrix

Assume for the moment that the goal of a test is to differentiate between a cochlear and a retrocochlear source of auditory impairment. Assume also that the test has only two outcomes: positive, predicting retrocochlear site; and negative, predicting cochlear site. Finally, assume that your patient has either a pure cochlear or a pure retrocochlear disorder. If there are two possible test results and two possible pathological states, the relationship of predicted to actual states can be displayed on a 2 × 2 matrix, as shown in Table 11-1.

Table 11–1.   Site of Disorder

Test Outcome	Retrocochlear	Cochlear	Total
Positive	Hit (HT)	False alarm (FA)	# Positive
Negative	Miss (MS)	Correct rejection (CR)	# Negative
TOTAL	# RE	# CE	

If the test result is positive and the patient truly has a retro-cochlear disorder, the outcome is called a *hit (HT)*. The ability of a test to identify a disorder that is actually present is called its *sensitivity*. If the test result is negative and the patient truly is free from retrocochlear disorder, the outcome is called a *correct rejection (CR);* the hypothesis of a retrocochlear site has been rightly rejected. The ability of a test to give a negative result when the patient is free of the condition of interest is called its *specificity*. High sensitivity and specificity are desirable attributes of a test, and lead to correct decisions.

Under ideal circumstances a test would have 100 percent sensitivity and 100 percent specificity; under actual circumstances this is never true of auditory tests. Predictive errors occur in two directions: First, a test result may be positive when the patient's impairment is cochlear; this is called a *false alarm (FA)*. Second, the test result may be negative when the disorder is actually retrocochlear; this outcome is called a *miss (MS)*. As errors, the miss and the false alarm lead to incorrect decisions and thus reduce the usefulness of a test in a clinical decision making.

The sensitivity of a test (percent) is determined by calculating the ratio of hits to the total number of patients having the disease, or

$$\text{Sensitivity} = [\text{HT} / (\text{HT} + \text{MS})] \times 100$$

Therefore, if 125 patients with retrocochlear disorder were tested and 70 had positive results, the sensitivity of the test would be [70/ (70 + 55)] × 100 = 56 percent. If the chance sensitivity or specificity of a test is 50 percent (i.e., that expected randomly or with guessing), the foregoing test would provide very little diagnostic advantage over guessing at the nature of the disorder by basing guesses on, for example, the patient's height or eye color.

Similarly, the specificity of a test is represented by the ratio of correct rejections to the total of disease-free patients:

$$\text{Specificity} = [\text{CR}/(\text{FA} + \text{CR})] \times 100$$

In this case, if 125 patients with cochlear disorder were tested and 95 obtained negative results, the test specificity would be [95/(30 + 95)] × 100 = 76 percent. Because HT + MS = 100 percent and CR + FA = 100 percent, we need only calculate HT and FA to determine the values of the other two terms.

Sensitivity and specificity vary inversely; that is, high sensitivity can be purchased only at the expense of a correspondingly high false alarm rate, and high specificity carries with it the disadvantage of a high miss rate. Furthermore, the HT and FA rates are determined not only by the details of the test, but also by the criterion set to call a result positive or negative. If the criterion changes, its sensitivity and specificity can be expected to change as well.

The Decision Axis

For purposes of this part of the discussion we have accepted an assumption (which is probably unwarranted in actual practice) that the scores achieved on a given test are normally distributed and have equal variance in two groups of subjects. One group has cochlear disorder, the other has retrocochlear disorder. In Figure 11–21, the probability of achieving a particular test score is plotted for the two groups. Notice that although the test scores achieved by the cochlear group are generally higher than those achieved by the retrocochlear group, there is an area of overlap in the two functions. This is the region of uncertainty, where errors in interpretation are likely to occur. The clinician is faced with the problem of deciding what test score will represent the boundary between positive and negative. The decision is made by considering the consequences—in terms of both costs and benefits—of certain errors. A boundary (or decision axis) placed at score X will provide high specificity, but it will also carry a high miss rate for patients with retrocochlear disorders who achieve scores on the high end of the retrocochlear distribution. Conversely, a decision axis placed at point Y will make the test very sensitive to retrocochlear disorders but will, at the same time, falsely identify a substantial number of patients who actually have cochlear problems.

What would be the consequences of errors made in each direction? A decision axis placed at point X would have the *benefit* of reducing the number of patients with cochlear disorders who might have to bear unnecessary financial expense, mental anguish, or physical risks of other diagnostic studies. The *cost*, however, would be that fewer retrocochlear disorders would be identified at an early stage, when chances of preserving hearing, vestibular function, and

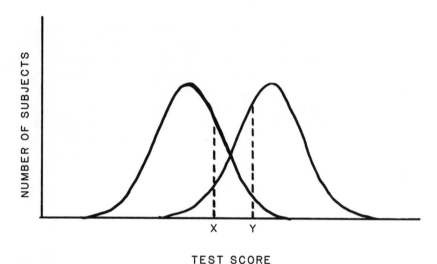

TEST SCORE

Figure 11–21. Distributions of test scores for two populations of listeners, one with cochlear disorder (right curve) and one with retrocochlear disorder (left curve). Note area of overlapping scores between the two groups. If all scores lower than score X are interpreted as a retrocochlear sign, the test will have high specificity, but a high miss rate as well. If the decision axis is placed at score Y, however, the test will have high sensitivity to retrocochlear disorders, but will also have a high false positive rate.

facial function after surgery are greatest. A decision axis placed at point Y has the *benefit* of early identification of retrocochlear disorders, but the *cost* is a substantial false alarm rate as well, resulting in the previously mentioned expense and risk factors and patient anxiety. A high false alarm rate also has the potential to reduce the diagnostic credibility of the clinician—a "cry wolf" effect.

Calculation of Posterior Probabilities

The foregoing method of calculating test sensitivity and specificity can yield completely accurate results only when the total number of patients with cochlear or retrocochlear disorder is verified; thus, it is not useful as a predictive device. In most clinical situations the cause of a disorder is unknown at the time of the testing. In these cases, the crucial question is, "What is the probability that a retrocochlear dysfunction actually exists when a positive test result is obtained?" That question can be answered by calculating the posterior probabilities, or the probability that the test is correct. Viewed another way, the measures of test performance—HT, FA, MS, CR—hold the nature of the disorder constant and calculate the probability of a positive or negative test result. For example, the correct rejection rate is the probability of obtaining a negative test result, given a cochlear disorder (Pr[– /CE]). The posterior probabilities that correspond to measures of test performance hold the test result constant and calculate the probability that it has correctly identified the disorder of interest. In this case, we would assess the probability of a cochlear disorder given a negative test result (Pr[CE/ –]). Four posterior probabilities can be calculated:

1. Pr[RE/ +] The probability that a retrocochlear disorder is present with a positive result
2. Pr[RE/ –] The probability that a retrocochlear disorder is present with a negative result
3. Pr[CE/ –] The probability that a cochlear disorder is present with a negative result
4. Pr[CE/ +] The probability that a cochlear disorder is present with a positive result

Probabilities 1 and 3 correspond to HT and CR, respectively; probabilities 2 and 4 correspond to MS and FA, respectively.

The measures of test performance would be useful in projecting the clinical utility of some test by calculating the HT and FA rates in one group of subjects known to have retrocochlear disorder and in another group known to be free of it. If there are equal numbers of subjects in each group, the prevalence of retrocochlear disorder is equal to the prevalence of cochlear disorder in the test "population."

In the clinic, however, the audiologist is faced with patients who are drawn from the general population in which the prevalence of retrocochlear disorders is much smaller, ranging from a possible high of 10 percent (Bauch, Rose, and Harner, 1982) to a more realistic estimate of 5 percent (Hart and Davenport, 1981) in patients who are suspected of having the disorder. In some clinical settings, the prevalence of retrocochlear disorders may be considerably lower than 5 percent, and in others it may be appreciably higher.

Posterior probabilities are calculated by applying a weighting factor of disease prevalence (Pd) in the general population to measures of test performance derived from a limited sample. Thus,

$$Pr[RE/+] = \cfrac{1}{1 + \cfrac{(FA)(1-Pd)}{(HT)(Pd)}}$$

$$Pr[RE/-] = \cfrac{1}{1 + \cfrac{(1-HT)(1-Pd)}{(1-FA)(Pd)}}$$

$$\Pr[CE/-1] = \cfrac{1}{1 + \cfrac{(1-HT)\,(Pd)}{(1-FA)\,(1-Pd)}}$$

$$\Pr[CE/+] = \cfrac{1}{1 + \cfrac{(HT)\,(Pd)}{(FA)\,(1-Pd)}}$$

The influence of disease prevalence can be made more clear by using some examples. First, consider a test with the characteristics of 60 percent HT and 15 percent FA. If the prevalence of retrocochlear disease is 5 percent, $\Pr[RE/+]$ would be

$$\cfrac{1}{1 + \cfrac{(0.15)\,(1-0.05)}{(0.6)\,(0.05)}}$$

$$\cfrac{1}{1 + \cfrac{(0.1425)}{(0.03)}}$$

$$\cfrac{1}{5.75}$$

$$\Pr[RE/+] \quad = \quad 0.17\ (17\%)$$

With this test, the probability that a retrocochlear disorder actually exists when the test is positive is only 17 percent; it would be incorrect (i.e., give a false alarm) 83 percent of the time! Contrast that outcome with the meaning of a negative result, again assuming a 5 percent retrocochlear prevalence:

$$\Pr[CE/-] \quad = \quad \cfrac{1}{1 + \cfrac{(1-0.60)\,(0.05)}{(1-0.15)\,(1-0.05)}}$$

$$= \quad \cfrac{1}{1 + \cfrac{0.02}{0.8075}}$$

$$= \quad \cfrac{1}{1.025}$$

$$= \quad 98\%$$

In this case, a negative test result is by far the more reliable indicant of the nature of the disorder. That is, you would be incorrect 83 percent of the time if you identified a retrocochlear disorder on the basis of a positive result on this test, but you would be incorrect only 2 percent of the time if you said a negative result ruled out a retrocochlear disorder.

How much would a more sensitive test (i.e., one with a higher HT) change the posterior probabilities? Assume that we had a superlative test, such as the ABR, with HT of 95 percent and FA of 5 percent:

$$\Pr[RE/+] = \cfrac{1}{1 + \cfrac{(0.05)(1 - 0.05)}{(0.95)(0.05)}}$$

$$= \cfrac{1}{1 + \cfrac{0.0475}{0.0475}}$$

$$= \frac{1}{2}$$

$$= 50\%$$

On the other hand:

$$\Pr[CE/-] = \cfrac{1}{1 + \cfrac{(1 - 0.95)(0.05)}{(1 - 0.05)(1 - 0.05)}}$$

$$= \cfrac{1}{1 + \cfrac{0.0025}{0.9025}}$$

$$= \frac{1}{1.00277}$$

$$= 99\%$$

Even with this very sensitive test, the probability of being wrong with a positive test result is still 50 percent. These examples illustrate the principle that *the lower the disease prevalence, the lower are the chances of being correct with a positive test result.* Therefore, the traditional language used in medical diagnosis, "Rule out x disease" serves as a reminder that negative test results may be more useful than positive test results when seeking to identify uncommon disorders.

Clinical Decision Analysis and the Test Battery

The procedures just described are used to assess the effectiveness of single tests. However, the introduction to this book argued for the necessity of a battery of tests and the cross-check principle in auditory assessment. How is the information provided by clinical decision analysis affected by using a test battery?

Assume a battery composed of three tests, A, B, and C. The individual sensitivity and specificity of these three tests are shown in Table 11-2.

The results of a test battery can be interpreted using either of two approaches: a "lax" (parallel) approach; or a "strict" (serial) approach (Jerger and Jerger, 1983). In the lax approach, the test battery is considered positive for retrocochlear disorder if any of the three tests are positive. Table 11-3 shows that as the number of tests in a battery increases, the sensitivity of the battery also increases. Notice also that the cost of the increased sensitivity is a decreased specificity; that is, there are more opportunities for false alarms. As the false alarm rate goes up and the disease prevalence remains low, the posterior probability Pr[RE/+] becomes even lower.

Now consider the results of a test battery interpreted using a strict criterion (one in which each component of the battery must be positive in order to consider the result indicative of retrocochlear dysfunction). As Table 11-4 demonstrates, such an approach decreases the sensitivity of the battery (relative to individual test sensitivity), but specificity is improved.

In this case, the opportunity for false alarms is reduced; thus, the probability of correctly ruling out retrocochlear disorder becomes much greater. It would appear, then, on the basis of these data and the calculation of posterior probabilities for a relatively low (5 percent) prevalence of retrocochlear disorders, that a strict approach to test battery interpretation improves the ability to rule out retrocochlear disorder. To paraphrase Jerger and Jerger (1983), the posterior probability Pr[CA/−] is not so much evidence for cochlear disorder as it is evidence *against* retrocochlear disorder.

SUMMARY

Clinical decision analysis is a quantifiable aid to interpretation of test results. It can be used to assess the efficiency of different tests, although not necessarily to rank order their clinical utility. The

Table 11-2.   Sensitivity and Specificity of a Test Battery

Test	Sensitivity	Specificity
A	85%	70%
B	65%	90%
C	85%	70%

sensitivity of a test is its ability to yield a positive result when a disorder of interest is present; test specificity means the ability of the test to produce a negative result when the subject is free of the disorder. Sensitivity and specificity vary inversely, and their values can be changed by criteria that are used to define "positive" or "negative" test results. The predictive value of a test can be assessed by determining posterior probabilities, which requires some knowledge of the prevalence of the target disorder in the population being tested. When the prevalence is low, negative test results are far more reliable in ruling out the disorder than are positive results at identifying the disorder. A test battery approach increases sensitivity if a "lax" interpretation criterion is used, but it increases specificity with a strict criterion. The latter approach is probably the desirable one in a situation in which the prevalence of the target disorder is low.

REAL WORLD CONSIDERATIONS

The previous chapters have described multiple tests that can be used to cross-validate each other and to meet the goals of the assessment. The issue, as it applied to "real world" situations, is *how many* of these procedures should be used in any given test situation. The answer to this issue is shaped by three factors: the presenting problem of the patient, the time constraints of the clinical situation, and how sure of the interpretation you want to be. Each of these factors can be further related to the cross-check principle.

Presenting Problem

The number and types of tests chosen for the test battery varies with the purpose of the assessment. At one end of the continuum, consider a patient who has come for assessment after middle ear surgery 2 to 3 weeks earlier. In this case, complete preoperative results

Table 11–3. Effects of a Lax Criterion on Sensitivity and Specificity

Test Positive	Sensitivity	Specificity
A	85%	70%
A or B	90%	65%
A or B or C	100%	55%

are usually available. The purpose of the evaluation is to determine how much hearing has been improved by the surgery. Here the test battery might be limited to pure tone A/C and B/C audiometry on the operated ear; the air conduction is compared with preoperative sensitivity, and the bone conduction would determine whether the cochlear reserve has changed. A spondee threshold would then be established to cross-check the pure tone results. If the surgery has involved work in the area of the oval or round windows, or if bone conduction sensitivity has worsened, the test battery would be expanded to include word identification measures. Immittance measures would not be completed so soon after middle ear surgery. On the other end of the continuum, consider the patient who is referred for evaluation with a history of vertigo, recent onset of tinnitus, or unilateral hearing loss. In this case, a test battery would include tests that could be used to differentiate between cochlear and retrocochlear types of disorders. Several cross-checks would be desirable: Pure tone sensitivity would establish the meaning of acoustic reflex patterns; performance-intensity functions for PB words and SSI materials would cross-check the audiogram configuration and allow you to determine whether the PB-SSI discrepancy could be accounted for by peripheral factors.

Time Constraints

There is no question that administering several tests takes more time than administering one or two. The clinician should consider, however, the quality and reliability of test information as a function of the time required to complete the test. For example, immittance measurement, in practiced hands, takes less time than traditional masked bone conduction audiometry, is subject to fewer extrinsic sources of variance and error, and provides information about the mechanical status of the middle ear (i.e., abnormally high or low stiffness) that cannot be inferred from the size of the air-bone gap. Acoustic reflex abnormalities such as elevated thresholds or adaptation suggest retrocochlear involvement that may have been unsus-

Table 11-4.   Effect of Using a Strict Criterion on Sensitivity and Specificity

Test Positive	Sensitivity	Specificity
A	85%	70%
A and B	60%	95%
A and B and C	55%	100%

pected. Pure tone air conduction thresholds alone convey nothing about the nature or site of auditory disorders but are crucial for the interpretation of physiological test results such as acoustic reflexes and ABR. A word identification test administered at a single suprathreshold level takes about 2 minutes per ear, but provides no unique information unless the score is unaccountably poor with respect to the audiogram. An audiologist working in a busy physician's office or clinic can schedule patients whose evaluations require long testing time for times when the physician is in surgery or making rounds. Another consideration should be the overall characteristics of the patient population encountered in your practice: An audiologist working with a neuro-otologist will expect to come into contact with more patients having retrocochlear dysfunction than would an audiologist who works in an educational setting, where the prevalence of middle ear disorders is higher. The objection that a test battery takes too much time is usually one that is offered by the *audiologist;* few *patients* would object to spending more time on a series of tests while the question about the nature of a disorder that will affect his or her life is thoroughly investigated.

Accountability and the Cross-check Principle

As noted earlier in the book, the test battery approach and the cross-check principle have been used successfully in medicine and other health care professions for some time. Most of us, for example, have had thorough physical examinations either on a routine basis or for a specific health complaint. During these examinations, a blood sample is often taken. The sample is then subjected to *multiple* tests that can provide information about many aspects of body function. There may be no suspicion, for example, that liver dysfunction is present, but a test for liver function is included in the blood test battery. In this way, a pattern of results that spans the physical examination, history, laboratory tests, and other tests such as x-ray films or electrocardiograms is established, complete with many internal cross-checks. The cross-checks not only establish what the disorder *is*, they clearly establish what it *is not*. Neither the physician nor the patient would be likely to consider that one or two tests are sufficient evidence to be sure of a diagnosis.

There is no reason to believe that a lesser standard of accountability for results should be applied to hearing assessment, an area closely related to an individual's ability to communicate successfully. The question of accountability (and its associated factor, liability) is a serious one. The importance of the test battery approach in general, and the cross-check principle in particular, is related to how important it is for you to be sure of your results. If the clinician will not be held accountable or liable for his or her results, a temptation can arise to simply follow orders and pass the results—and the responsibility—along to a higher level. This approach, although stress-free, does nothing to enhance the audiologist's image as a hearing health professional.

Your well-informed choices in these matters, therefore, influence your status as a clinician, your patients' lives, and the quality of clinical assessment of auditory function.

STUDY QUESTIONS

1. Distinguish between sensitivity and specificity.
2. How does disease prevalence influence the accuracy of test interpretation?
3. Why would a "strict" interpretation criterion be more consistent with the cross-check principle?

SUGGESTED READINGS

Principles of Immittance

Bennett, M. (1984). Impedance concepts relating to the acoustic reflex. In S. Silman (Ed.), *The Acoustic Reflex* (pp. 36–61). New York: Academic Press.

Berlin, C., and Cullen, J. (1980). Physical basis of impedance measurement. In J. Jerger and J. Northern (Eds.), *Clinical Impedance Audiometry* (pp. 83–108). Acton, MA: American Electromedics Corp.

Margolis, R. (1981). Fundamentals of acoustic immittance. In G. Popelka (Ed.), *Hearing Assessment with the Acoustic Reflex* (pp. 117–143). New York: Grune & Stratton.

Møller, A. (1965). An experimental study of the acoustic impedance of the middle ear and its transmission properties. *Acta Otolaryngologica, 58,* 129–149.

Popelka, G. (1981). Instrumentation and procedures for measuring acoustic reflex thresholds. In G. Popelka (Ed.), *Hearing Assessment with the Acoustic Reflex* (pp. 47–58). New York: Grune & Stratton.

Wiley, T., and Block, M. (1985). Overview and basic principles of acoustic immittance measurements. In J. Katz (Ed.), *Handbook of Clinical Audiology* (3rd ed.) (pp. 423–437). Baltimore: Williams & Wilkins.

Zwislocki, J. (1963). An acoustic method for clinical examination of the ear. *J. Speech Hear. Res., 6,* 303–314.

Clinical Applications of Immittance

Anderson, S. (1976). The intratympanic muscles. In R. Hinchcliffe and D. Harrison (Eds.), *Scientific Foundations of Otolaryngology* (pp. 257–280). London: Wm. Heinemann Medical Books, Ltd.

Borg, E. (1968). A quantitative study of the effect of the acoustic stapedius reflex on sound transmission through the middle ear of man. *Acta Otolaryngol, 60,* 461–472.

Brooks, D. (1969). The use of the electroacoustic impedance bridge in the assessment of middle ear function. *Int. Audiol., 8,* 563–569.

Feldman, A. (1976). Tympanometry: application and interpretation. *Ann. Otol. Rhinol. Laryngol* (Suppl. 25), 202–208.

Gelfand, S., and Piper, N. (1984). Acoustic reflex thresholds: variability and distribution effects. *Ear Hear., 5,* 228–234.

Hayes, D., and Jerger, J. (1983). Signal-averaging of the acoustic reflex: Diagnostic applications of amplitude characteristics. *Scand. Audiol.* (Suppl. 17), 31–36.

Jerger, J., and Hayes, D. (1980). Diagnostic applications of impedance audiometry. Middle ear disorder; sensorineural disorder. In J. Jerger and J. Northern (Eds.), *Clinical Impedance Audiometry* (pp. 109–127). Acton, MA: American Electromedics Corp.

Northern, J. (1980). Clinical measurement procedures in impedance audiometry. In J. Jerger and J. Northern (Eds.), *Clinical Impedance Audiometry* (pp. 19–39). Acton, MA: American Electromedics Corp.

Popelka, G. (1981). Instrumentation and procedures for measuring acoustic reflex thresholds. In G. Popelka (Ed.), *Hearing Assessment with the Acoustic Reflex* (pp. 47–58). New York: Grune & Stratton.

Popelka, G. (1981). The acoustic reflex in normal and pathological ears. In G. Popelka (Ed.), *Hearing Assessment with the Acoustic Reflex* (pp. 5–21). New York: Grune & Stratton.

Silman, S. (1984). *The Acoustic Reflex. Basic Principles and Clinical Applications.* New York: Academic Press.

Terkildsen, K. (1976). Pathologies and their effect on middle ear function. In A. Feldman and L. Wilber (Eds.), *Acoustic Impedance and Admittance* (pp. 78–102). Baltimore: Williams & Wilkins.

Pure Tone Audiometry

Berlin, C. (1970). *Programmed Instruction in the Decibel in Clinical Audiology.* New Orleans: Kresge Hearing Research Laboratory, Louisiana State University School of Medicine.

Davis, H., and Kranz, F. (1964). The international standard reference zero for pure tone audiometers and its relation to the evaluation of impairment of hearing. *J. Speech Hear. Res., 7,* 7–14.

Dirks, D. (1978). Bone conduction testing. In J. Katz (Ed.), *Handbook of Clinical Audiology* (2nd ed., pp. 110–123). Baltimore: Williams & Wilkins.

Goldstein, D., and Hayes, C. (1965). The occlusion effect in bone conduction hearing. *J. Speech Hear. Res., 8,* 137–148.

Principles of Masking

Jerger, J. (1971). Principles and limitations of the Rainville methodology. *Audiology, 10,* 129–137.

Naunton, R. (1962). The masking dilemma in bilateral conduction deafness. *Arch. Otolaryngol., 72,* 753–757.

Sanders, J. (1978). Masking. In J. Katz (Ed.), *Handbook of Clinical Audiology* (2nd ed.). Baltimore: Williams & Wilkins.

Studebaker, G. (1967). Clinical masking of the non-test ear. *J. Speech Hear. Dis., 32,* 360–371.

Speech Audiometry

Chaiklin, J. (1959). The relation among three selected auditory speech thresholds. *J. Speech Hear. Res., 2,* 237–243.

Dillon, H. (1982). A quantitative examination of the sources of speech discrimination test score variability. *Ear Hear., 3,* 51–58.

Dubno, J., and Dirks, D. (1983). Suggestions for optimizing reliability with the Synthetic Sentence Identification test. *J. Speech Hear. Dis., 48,* 98–103.

Jerger, J. (1970). Diagnostic significance of speech test procedures utilizing phonetically balanced words. In C. Rojskjaer (Ed.), *Speech Audiometry* (pp. 91–101). Odense, Denmark: Andelbogtrykkeriet.

Jerger, S., and Jerger, J. (1979). Quantifying auditory handicap. A new approach. *Audiology, 18,* 225–237.

Marshall, L., and Bacon, S. (1981). Prediction of speech discrimination scores from audiometric data. *Ear Hear., 2,* 148–155.

Rupp, R., and Stockdell, K. (1980). *Speech Protocols in Audiology.* New York: Grune & Stratton.

Tobin, H. (1978). Disordered functions approach to audiologic diagnosis. In S. Singh and J. Lynch (Eds.), *Diagnostic Procedures in Hearing, Speech, and Language* (pp. 57–103). Baltimore: University Park Press.

Wilson, R., Morgan, D., and Dirks, D. (1973). A proposed SRT procedure and its statistical precedent. *J. Speech Hear. Dis., 30,* 184–191.

REFERENCES

American National Standards Institute. (1970). *Specifications for audiometers.* (ANSI S3.6-1969). New York: American National Standards Institute, Inc.

American Speech and Hearing Association, Committee on Audiometric Evaluation (1974). Guidelines for audiometric symbols, *ASHA, 17,* 260–264.

Arlen, H. (1977). The otomandibular syndrome: a new concept. *Ear, Nose, and Throat J., 6,* 36–37.

Bauch, C., and Robinette, M. (1978). Alcohol and the acoustic reflex: effects of stimulus spectrum, subject variability, and sex. *J. Am. Aud. Soc., 4,* 104–112.

Bauch, C., Rose, D., and Harner, S. (1982). Auditory brain stem response results from 255 patients with suspected retrocochlear involvement. *Ear Hear., 3,* 83–86.

Berlin, C. (1982). Ultra-audiometric hearing in the hearing impaired and the use of upward-shifting hearing aids. *Volta Rev., 84,* 352–363.

Berlin, C., and Cullen, J. (1980). Physical basis of impedance measurement. In J. Jerger and J. Northern (Eds.), *Clinical Impedance Audiometry* (2nd ed.) (pp. 1–18). Acton, MA: American Electromedics Corp.

Bluestone, C. (1976). Assessment of eustachian tube function. In J. Jerger and J. Northern (Eds.), *Clinical Impedance Audiometry* (pp. 83–108). Acton, MA: American Electromedics.

Bocca, E., and Calearo, C. (1963). Central hearing processes. In J. Jerger (Ed.), *Modern Developments in Audiology* (1st ed.) (pp. 337–370). New York: Academic Press.

Borg, E. (1973). On the neuronal organization of the acoustic middle ear reflex. A physiological and anatomical study. *Brain Res., 49,* 101–123.

Borg, E., and Møller, A. (1968). The effect of ethylalcohol and pentobarbitol sodium on the acoustic reflex in man. *Acta Otolaryngol., 64,* 415–426.

Borg, E., and Zakrisson, J. (1973). Stapedius reflex and speech features. *J. Acoust. Soc. Am., 54,* 525–527.

Brooks, D. (1976). Acoustic impedance. In R. Hinchcliffe and D. Harrison (Eds.), *Scientific Foundations of Otolaryngology* (pp. 282–290). London: Wm. Heinemann Medical Books, Ltd.

Carhart, R., and Jerger, J. (1959). Preferred method for clinical determination of pure tone thresholds. *J. Speech Hear. Dis., 24,* 330–345.

Dorman, M., Cedar, I., Hannley, M., Leek, M., and Lindholm, J. M. (in press). Influence of the acoustic reflex on vowel recognition. *J. Speech Hear. Res.*

Dorman, M., and Hannley, M. (1985). Identification of speech and speech-like signals by hearing impaired listeners. In R. Daniloff (Ed.), *Speech Science. Recent Advances* (pp. 111–153). San Diego: College-Hill Press.

Downs, D., and Crum, M. (1980). The hyperactive acoustic reflex. *Arch. Otolaryngol., 106*, 401–404.

Gelfand, S. (1984). The contralateral acoustic-reflex threshold. In S. Silman (Ed.), *The Acoustic Reflex* (pp. 138–187). Orlando, FL: Academic Press.

Gelfand, S., and Silman, S. (1982). Acoustic reflex thresholds in brain-damaged patients. *Ear Hear., 3*, 93–95.

Goodhill, V., Dirks, D., and Malmquist, C. (1970). Bone conduction thresholds: relationships of frontal and mastoid measurements in conductive hypacusis. *Arch. Otolaryngol., 91*, 250–256.

Hannley, M., and Jerger, J. (1981). PB rollover and the acoustic reflex. *Audiology, 20*, 251–258.

Hart, R., and Davenport, J. (1981). Diagnosis of acoustic neuroma. *Neurosurgery, 9*, 450–463.

Hawkins, J., and Stevens, S. (1950). Masking of pure tones and of speech by white noise. *J. Acoust. Soc. Am, 22*, 6–13.

Hodgson, W. (1980). *Basic Audiologic Evaluation.* Baltimore: Williams & Wilkins.

Hood, J. (1960). The principles and practice of bone conduction audiometry. *Laryngoscope, 70*, 1211–1228.

Jerger, J. (1970). Clinical experience with impedance audiometry. *Arch. Otolaryngol., 92*, 311–324.

Jerger, J. (1976). A proposed audiometric symbol system for scholarly publications. *Arch. Otolaryng., 102*, 33–36.

Jerger, J., Anthony, L., Jerger, S., and Crump, B. (1974). Studies in impedance audiometry: III Middle ear disorders. *Arch. Otolaryngol., 99*, 165–171.

Jerger, J., Fifer, R., Jenkins, H., and Mecklenburg, D. (in press). Stapedial reflex to electrical stimulation in a patient with cochlear implant. *Annals of Otol., Rhinol., Laryngol.*

Jerger, J., and Hayes, D. (1976). The crosscheck principle in pediatric audiology. *Arch. Otolaryng., 102*, 614–620.

Jerger, J., and Hayes, D. (1977). Diagnostic speech audiometry. *Arch. Otolaryngol., 103*, 216–222.

Jerger, J., and Jerger, S. (1971). Diagnostic significance of PB word functions. *Arch. Otolaryngol., 93*, 573–580.

Jerger, J., Speaks, C., and Trammell, J. (1968). A new approach to speech audiometry. *J. Speech Hear. Dis., 33*, 318–328.

Jerger, J., and Tillman, T. (1960). A new method for the clinical determination of sensorineural acuity level (SAL). *Arch. Otolaryngol., 71*, 948–953.

Jerger, J., Weikers, N., Sharbrough, F., and Jerger, S. (1969). Bilateral lesions of the temporal lobe. *Acta Otolaryngol.* (Suppl. 258).

Jerger, S., and Jerger, J. (1977). Diagnostic value of crossed vs. uncrossed acoustic reflexes. Eighth nerve and brain stem disorders. *Arch. Otolaryngol., 103*, 445–453.

Jerger, S., and Jerger, J. (1981). *Auditory Disorders: A Manual for Clinical Evaluation.* Boston: Little, Brown, Co.

Jerger, S., and Jerger, J. (1983). Evaluation of diagnostic audiometric tests. *Audiology, 22,* 144–161.

Lilly, D. (1973). Measurement of acoustic impedance at the tympanic membrane. In J. Jerger (Ed.), *Modern Developments in Audiology.* (pp. 345–406). New York: Academic Press.

Lyregaard, P., Robinson, D., and Hinchcliffe, R. (1976). A feasibility study of diagnostic speech audiometry. *National Physical Laboratory Acoustics Report* AC 73.

McCandless, G., and Goering, D. (1974). Changes in loudness after stapedectomy. *Arch. Otolaryngol., 100,* 344–350.

McCandless, G., and Schumacher, M. (1979). Auditory dysfunction with facial paralysis. *Arch. Otolaryngol., 105,* 271–274.

Miller, M. (1985). The integration of audiologic findings. In J. Katz (Ed.), *Handbook of Clinical Audiology* (3rd ed.) (pp. 259–272). Baltimore: Williams & Wilkins.

Newman, B., and Fanger, L. (1973). *Otoadmittance Handbook 2.* Concord, MA: Grason-Stadler, Inc.

Rainville, M. (1959). New method of masking for the determination of bone conduction curves. *Transl. Beltone Inst. for Hearing Res., 11,* July.

Rosenberg, P. (1978). Case history: The first test. In J. Katz (Ed.), *Handbook of Clinical Audiology* (2nd ed.) (pp. 77–80). Baltimore: Williams & Wilkins.

Rupp, R. (1980). Classical approaches to the determination of the spondee threshold. In R. Rupp and K. Stockdell (Eds.), *Speech Protocols in Audiology* (pp. 67–97). New York: Grune & Stratton.

Speaks, C., and Jerger, J. (1965). Method for the measurement of speech identification. *J. Speech Hear. Res., 8,* 185–194.

Speaks, C., Jerger, J., and Jerger, S. (1966). Performance-intensity characteristics of synthetic sentences. *J. Speech Hear. Res., 9,* 305–312.

Studebaker, G. (1962). Placement of vibrator in bone conduction testing. *J. Speech Hear. Res., 5,* 321–331.

Thomas, W., Preslar, M., Summers, R., and Stewart, J. (1969). Calibration and working condition of 100 audiometers. *Public Health Rep., 84,* 311–327.

Thompson, G. (1983). Structure and function of the central auditory system. *Seminars in Hearing, 4,* 81–96.

Tobin, H. (1978). Disordered functions approach to audiologic diagnosis. In S. Singh and J. Lynch (Eds.), *Diagnostic Procedures in Hearing, Speech, and Language* (pp. 57–103). Baltimore: University Park Press.

Tonndorf, J. (1966). Bone conduction; studies in experimental animals. *Acta Otolaryngol.* (Suppl. 213), 1–32.

Tonndorf, J. (1972). Bone conduction. In J. Tobias (Ed.), *Foundations of Modern Auditory Theory* (pp. 195–237). New York: Academic Press.

Turner, R., and Nielsen, D. (1984). Application of clinical decision analysis to audiological tests. *Ear Hear., 5,* 125–132.

Wilber, L. (1985). Calibration: Puretone, speech, and noise signals. In J. Katz (Ed.), *Handbook of Clinical Audiology* (3rd ed.) (pp. 116–150). Baltimore: Williams & Wilkins.

Wilson, R., Shanks, J., and Lilly, D. (1984). Acoustic-reflex adaptation. In S.

Silman (Ed.), *The Acoustic Reflex* (pp. 329–387). Orlando, FL: Academic Press.

Zwislocki, J. (1963). An acoustic method for clinical examination of the ear. *J. Speech Hear. Res., 6,* 303–314.

Author Index

Subject Index

A

ABR. *See* Auditory brain stem response
Accountability, 2, 219–220
Acoustic reflex, 65–86
  abnormalities, 70–71
  biological preconditions for, 71–72
  characteristics, 66–72
  contralateral, 68, 73
  effect of hearing impairment on, 70, 79, 82, 187–188, 199
  effect on sound transmission, 65
  ipsilateral, 68, 73
  mechanism, 65–66, 68–69
  nonpathological influences, 67
Adaptation, acoustic reflex, 70, 71
Admittance, 44–45
Air-bone gap, 98
  classifying audiograms and, 132–133, 181, 196, 205–206
  effect on acoustic reflex, 78–80
  masking dilemma and, 118
  mechanism, 98
Air conduction, 96–97
  threshold elevation, meaning, 135–136
Alcohol, effects on auditory function, 24
American National Standards Institute (ANSI), 8, 9, 12, 92, 93
  audiometric norms, 9, 94, 154
American Standards Association (ASA), 7, 9
  audiometric norms, 9

ANSI. *See* American National Standards Institute
ASA. *See* American Standards Association
Attenuator, linearity, 12, 143
Audiogram, 129–136
  classification of, 132–136
  description, 96, 97
  symbols for, 129–130
Audiometric zero, 92
  norms for, 94
Auditory brain stem response (ABR), 3, 209, 215
Aural habilitation, 4, 185, 191
Average, pure tone (PTA), 133
  relation to speech thresholds, 155–156

B

Battery, test, 1, 216, 217, 219, 220
  auditory assessment with, 2
  selecting components, 3
  time constraints with, 5, 218–219
Bone conduction, 97–101
  compressional, 99
  frequency dependency, 98–99
  inertial, 99
  mechanisms, 98–100
  necessity for testing, 84, 97, 109, 117, 186, 188, 205
  occlusion effect with, 99–100
  oscillator, placement of, 139
  relation to air conduction, 97